Lecture Notes in Computer Science 7330

Commenced Publication in 1973
Founding and Former Series Editors:
Gerhard Goos, Juris Hartmanis, and Jan van Leeuwen

W0227633

Editorial Board

David Hutchison
Lancaster University, UK

Takeo Kanade
Carnegie Mellon University, Pittsburgh, PA, USA

Josef Kittler
University of Surrey, Guildford, UK

Jon M. Kleinberg
Cornell University, Ithaca, NY, USA

Alfred Kobsa
University of California, Irvine, CA, USA

Friedemann Mattern
ETH Zurich, Switzerland

John C. Mitchell
Stanford University, CA, USA

Moni Naor
Weizmann Institute of Science, Rehovot, Israel

Oscar Nierstrasz
University of Bern, Switzerland

C. Pandu Rangan
Indian Institute of Technology, Madras, India

Bernhard Steffen
TU Dortmund University, Germany

Madhu Sudan
Microsoft Research, Cambridge, MA, USA

Demetri Terzopoulos
University of California, Los Angeles, CA, USA

Doug Tygar
University of California, Berkeley, CA, USA

Gerhard Weikum
Max Planck Institute for Informatics, Saarbruecken, Germany

Purang Abolmaesumi   Leo Joskowicz
Nassir Navab   Pierre Jannin (Eds.)

Information Processing in Computer-Assisted Interventions

Third International Conference, IPCAI 2012
Pisa, Italy, June 27, 2012
Proceedings

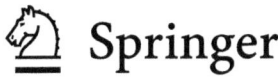 Springer

Volume Editors

Purang Abolmaesumi
The University of British Columbia
Department of Electrical and Computer Engineering
Vancouver, BC, V6T 1Z4, Canada
E-mail: purang@ece.ubc.ca

Leo Joskowicz
The Hebrew University of Jerusalem
School of Engineering and Computer Science, ELSC
Givat Ram, Jerusalem 91904, Israel
E-mail: josko@cs.huji.ac.il

Nassir Navab
Technische Universität München
Institut für Informatik I16
Boltzmannstr. 3, 85748 Garching, Germany
E-mail: navab@cs.tum.edu

Pierre Jannin
Inserm, Université de Rennes 1
MediCIS, UMR 1099 LTSI
2, Avenue du Pr. Léon Bernard, CS 34317, 35043 Rennes Cedex, France
E-mail: pierre.jannin@univ-rennes1.fr

ISSN 0302-9743   e-ISSN 1611-3349
ISBN 978-3-642-30617-4   e-ISBN 978-3-642-30618-1
DOI 10.1007/978-3-642-30618-1
Springer Heidelberg Dordrecht London New York

Library of Congress Control Number: 2012938254

CR Subject Classification (1998): I.6, I.4-5, J.3, I.2.10, I.3.5

LNCS Sublibrary: SL 6 – Image Processing, Computer Vision, Pattern Recognition,
and Graphics

Typesetting: Camera-ready by author, data conversion by Scientific Publishing Services, Chennai, India

Printed on acid-free paper

Springer is part of Springer Science+Business Media (www.springer.com)

Preface

Minimally invasive surgical interventions are one of the key drivers of the search for ways to use computer-based information technology to link preoperative planning and surgeon actions in the operating room. Computers, used in conjunction with advanced surgical assist devices, are influencing how procedures are currently performed.

Computer-assisted intervention (CAI) systems make it possible to carry out surgical interventions that are more precise and less invasive than conventional procedures, while recording all relevant data. This data logging, coupled with appropriate tracking of patient outcomes, is a key enabler for a new level of quantitative patient outcome assessment and treatment improvement. The goals of CAI systems are to enhance the dexterity, visual feedback, and information integration of the surgeon. While medical equipment is currently available to assist the surgeons in specific tasks, it is the synergy between these capabilities that gives rise to a new paradigm.

The Information Processing and Computer-Assisted Intervention (IPCAI) Conference was created as a forum to present the latest developments in CAI. The main technological focus is on patient-specific modeling and its use in interventions, image-guided and robotic surgery, real-time tracking and imaging. IPCAI aims at taking the particular aspects of interest and importance to CAI into account directly during the paper review process. IPCAI seeks papers presenting novel technical concepts, clinical needs and applications, as well as hardware, software, and systems and their validation.

The yearly IPCAI conferences were initiated in 2010 in Geneva, Switzerland, and the second in 2011 Berlin, Germany. This volume contains the proceedings of the Third IPCAI Conferencethat took place on June 27, 2012, in Pisa, Italy. This year, we received 31 full papers submissions, 15 from North America, 15 from Europe, and one from Asia. These submissions were reviewed by a total of 50 external reviewers, coordinated by 11 Program Committee members. A "primary" and "secondary" Program Committee member were assigned to each paper, and each paper received at least three external reviews. After the initial review process, the authors were given the opportunity to respond to the reviewers' and the Program Committee members' comments. Finally, an independent body of six Program Board members discussed all papers and a final decision was made, where 17 very high quality papers were accepted. The final submissions were re-reviewed by the Program Committee members to ensure that all reviewers' comments were addressed.

The format of the IPCAI conference allows more time for constructive discussion. In a departure from prior years, all authors of accepted papers were asked to give short five-minute platform presentations. These presentations were followed by two "interactive" poster sessions with organized discussion. Following this initial interaction, the conference delegates voted for a list of papers where they were interested in a longer platform presentation. For these papers, at least 30 minutes were allocated for questions from the attendees and the committee members.

We would like to take this opportunity to thank our fellow Area Chairs: Hervé Delingette, INRIA, France; Gabor Fichtinger, Queen's, Canada; Makoto Hashizume, Fukuoka, Japan; Thomas Langø, SINTEF, Norway; Ken Mahsamune, Tokyo, Japan; Lena Meier-Hein, DKFZ, Germany; Parvin Mousavi, Queen's, Canada; Sebastien Ourselin, UCL, UK; Graeme Penney, King's College, UK; Ziv Yaniv, Children's Hospital, USA, and Guoyan Zheng, University of Bern, Switzerland; and Program Board Members: David Hawkes, UCL, UK; Kensaku Mori, Nagoya, Japan; Tim Salcudean, UBC, Canada; Gabor Szekely, ETH, Switzerland; Russell Taylor, JHU, USA, and Guang-Zhong Yang, ICL, UK.

We would also like to thank all the authors that submitted their papers to IPCAI and for their subsequent work in revising the papers for final publication.

March 2012   Purang Abolmaesumi
                                                         Leo Joskowicz

Organization

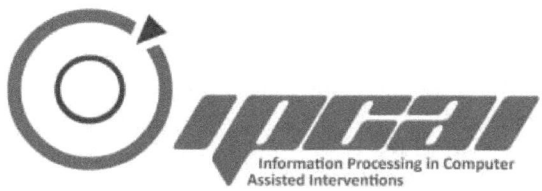

2012 Executive Committee

Program Chairs

Purang Abolmaesoumi   UBC, Canada
Leo Joskowicz   Hebrew University, Israel

General Chairs

Nassir Navab   CAMP/TUM, Germany
Pierre Jannin   INSERM, Rennes, France

Area Chairs

Hervé Delingette   INRIA, France
Gabor Fichtinger   Queen's University, Canada
Makoto Hashizume   Fukuoka, Japan
Thomas Langø   SINTEF, Norway
Ken Masamune   Tokyo, Japan
Lena Meier-Hein   DKFZ, Germany
Parvin Mousavi   Queen's University, Canada
Sebastien Ourselin   London, UK
Graeme Penney   King's College, UK
Ziv Yaniv   Georgetown, USA
Guoyan Zheng   University of Bern, Switzerland
Tim Salcudean   UBC, Canada
Ichiro Sakuma   University of Tokyo, Japan

Local Organization Chairs

Franziska Schweikert   CARS office, Germany
Stefanie Demirci   CAMP/TUM, Germany

Industrial Liaisons

Wolfgang Wein   White Lion Tech. GmbH, Germany
Ameet Jain   Philips, USA
Tom Vercauteren   Mauna Kea, France
Simon DiMaio   Intuitive Surgical, USA
Joerg Traub   SurgicEye, Germany
Leslie Holton   Medtronic, USA

IPCAI Steering Committee

Kevin Cleary   DC Children's Hospital, USA
Gabor Fichtinger   Queen's University, Canada
Makoto Hashizume   Fukuoka, Japan
Dave Hawkes   UCL, UK
Pierre Jannin   INSERM, Rennes, France
Leo Joskowicz   Hebrew University, Israel
Ron Kikinis   Boston, USA
Kensaku Mori   Nagoya University, Japan
Nassir Navab   CAMP/TUM, Germany
Terry Peters   London, Canada
Tim Salcudean   UBC, Canada
Gábor Székely   ETH, Switzerland
Russell Taylor   JHU, USA
Guang-Zhong Yang   Imperial College, UK

Reviewers

Ahmad Ahmadi	Gregory Hager	Hongen Liao
Paul Aljabar	Tatsuya Harada	Frank Lindseth
Wolfgang Birkfellner	Makoto Hashizume	Marius George
Oliver Burgert	Noby Hata	Linguraru
Jorge Cardoso	Joachim Hornegger	Lena Maier-Hein
Louis Collins	Mingxing Hu	Ken Masamune
Benoit Dawant	Satoshi Ieiri	Daniel Mirota
Herve Delingette	Ameet Jain	Peter Mountney
Eddie Edwards	Peter Kazanzides	Parvin Mousavi
Gabor Fichtinger	Andrew King	Sebastien Muller
Michael Figl	Takayuki Kitasaka	Ryoichi Nakamura
Moti Freiman	Thomas Lango	Stephane Nicolau

Lutz Nolte
Sebastien Ourselin
Nicolas Padoy
Srivatsan Pallavaram
Graeme Penney
Franjo Pernus
Terry Peters
Tobias Reichl
Kawal Rhode
Robert Rohling

Ruby Shamir
Luc Soler
Stefanie Speidel
Danail Stoyanov
Takashi Suzuki
Raphael Sznitman
Jocelyne Troccaz
Tamas Ungi
Theo van Walsum
Tom Vercauteren

Kirby Vosburgh
Lejing Wang
Stefan Weber
Wolfgang Wein
Yasushi Yamauchi
Guang-Zhong Yang
Ziv Yaniv
Guoyan Zheng

Table of Contents

Cardiac Applications

Neurosurgery, Surgical Workflow and Skill Evaluation

Template-Based Conformal Shape-from-Motion-and-Shading for Laparoscopy

Abed Malti, Adrien Bartoli, and Toby Collins

ALCoV-ISIT,
UMR 6284 CNRS/Université d'Auvergne,
28 Place Henri Dunant,
Clermont-Ferrand, France
http://isit.u-clermont1.fr/{~abed, ~ab, content/Toby-Collins}

Abstract. Shape-from-Shading (SfS) is one of the fundamental techniques to recover depth from a single view. Such a method has shown encouraging but limited
results in laparoscopic surgery due to the complex reflectance properties of the organ tissues. On the other hand, Template-Based Deformable-Shape-from-Motion
(DSfM) has been recently used to recover a coarse 3D shape in laparoscopy.
    We propose to combine both geometric and photometric cues to robustly re-
construct 3D human organs. Our method is dubbed Deformable-Shape-from-
Motion-and-Shading (DSfMS). It tackles the limits of classical SfS and DSfM
methods: First the photometric template is reconstructed using rigid SfM (Shape-
from-Motion) while the surgeon is exploring – but not deforming – the peritoneal
environment. Second a rough 3D deformed shape is computed using a recent
method for elastic surface from a single laparoscopic image. Third a fine 3D deformed shape is recovered using shading and specularities.
    The proposed approach has been validated on both synthetic data and in-vivo
laparoscopic videos of a uterus. Experimental results illustrate its effectiveness
compared to SfS and DSfM.

1   Introduction

Over the past few years efforts have been made to develop systems for computer aided
laparosurgery. It consists on helping the practitioners during the intervention to improve
their perception of the intra-operative environment [10]. 3D sensing offers a virtual
controllable view-point and is one of the major possible improvements to the current
technology. However, due to the unpredictable, complex and elastic behaviour of living
peritoneal tissues, 3D shape recovery from laparoscopic images is a difficult and open
problem.

On the one hand, DSfM methods has shown effectiveness in recovering 3D shapes
of elastic deformations in laparoscopy [17,7]. Based on how does the feature correspondences cover the surface, the 3D reconstruction can go from coarse to fine when
the correspondences go from sparse to dense. Usually human organs are textureless
and very specular which makes it difficult to densely cover the surface with feature
correspondences using automatic feature detection and matching. On the other hand,
SfS methods allow one to recover surface details. However, it is difficult to achieve
remarkable 3D reconstructions due to the complex reflectance of the organ tissues. In
addition, SfS does not allow one to solve temporal registration. In order to take advantage of these two methods and overcome their drawbacks, we propose to combine

P. Abolmaesumi et al. (Eds.): IPCAI 2012, LNAI 7330, pp. 1–10, 2012.

them in a Deformbale-Shape-from-Motion-and-Shading (DSfMS) framework. Figure 1 shows the effectiveness of our proposal when compared to SfS and DSfM: the shading cue provides details on the surface and the motion cue adds smoothness and global consistency.

Paper Organization. Section §2 presents state-of-the-art. Section §3 gives a geometric characterization of smooth surfaces. Section §4 presents the 3D template reconstruction. Section §5 gives a photometirc reconstruction of the template albedo map. Section §6 recalls monocular conformal reconstruction. Section §7 presents monocular conformal reconstruction with shading cues. We finally report experimental results in section §8 and conclude. Our notation will be introduced throughout the paper.

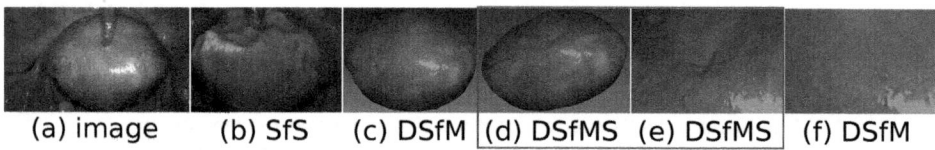

(a) image   (b) SfS   (c) DSfM |(d) DSfMS   (e) DSfMS| (f) DSfM

Fig. 1. Qualitative comparison between the proposed approach and previous methods. Using one Single input image with deformed organ from an in-vivo video sequence, the result of three reconstruction methods is shown. The reconstruction using classic SfS in figure (b) shows bumpy region. The reconstructions using DSfM and DSfMS in (c) and (d) show smoother results. An enlarged view of the deformed region allows us to observe in figure (e) that our DSfMS recovers the deformation while in figure (f) the DSfM recovers a coarse smooth surface.

2   Related Work

Intra-operative 3D sensing has recently gained a lot of interest in the field of laparosurgery. Various methods have been proposed that can be classified as active and passive. Active approaches consist of sensing techniques that modify the laparoscope's hardware. In [5,6] an approach based on the detection of a laser beam line is described. The approach requires the insertion of two monocular endoscopes: one for the projection of the laser beam and one for observing the projected laser beam. In [12] a prototype of Time-of-Flight (ToF) endoscope is proposed and in [19] a set of incremental algorithms for 3D reconstruction has shown promising results using ToF endoscopes. Passive approaches consist of vision techniques based only on 'regular' images from the laparoscope. Both stereo and monocular endoscopes are concerned. In [17,3] methods based on disparity map computation for stereo-laparoscope have been proposed. Visual SLAM for dense surface reconstruction has been proposed in [18]. In the context of monocular laparoscopy, very few methods were proposed [2].

However, the computer vision community has made some effective achievements in the domain of template-based monocular 3D reconstruction of deformable surfaces. Using a template-based method provides a full geometric description of the surface rather than just a sparse or partially dense description as in the previously cited methods. This allows one to render the surface from a new viewpoint, recover self-occluded parts, and opens applications based on Augmented Reality. The problem of template-based monocular 3D shape recovery is under-constrained because there is an infinite number of 3D surfaces that can project to the same image data. It is then of critical importance to constrain the problem to have a unique consistent solution or at least a small set of plausible solutions. Over the recent years, different types of physical and statistical constraints were proposed [8,15]. An important physical prior is isometry [1,13], which imposes that the geodesic distance is preserved by deformations. Recently a 3D conformal method has been proposed to reconstruct elastic deformations in the context of laparosurgery [7]. To provide good reconstruction results, SfM needs feature detection and matching in the deformed areas. The SfS problem is one of the eldest and fundamental problems in computer vision [23,14]. Recovering depths using shading cues has been extensively used for both rigid and deformable objects [23]. To provide good reconstruction results, SfS needs an estimation of the reflectance map of the reconstructed surface.

To overcome the bottleneck of SfS and DSfM, we can take advantage of both methods: using feature-based reconstruction to recover a deformed 3D surface and use shading cues to refine the reconstruction of areas which lack tracked features. This combined approach has been used in several other conditions to recover coarse to fine 3D shapes: For instance in rigid 3D reconstruction [22] presented an algorithm for computing optical flow, shape, motion, lighting, and albedo from an image sequence of a rigidly-moving Lambertian object under distant illumination. [20] proposed an approach to recover shape detail to dynamic scene geometry captured from multi-view video frames. [8] presented a closed-form solution to the problem of recovering the 3D shape of a non-rigid potentially stretchable surface from 3D-to-2D correspondences. In [16], a strategy for dense 3D depth recovery and temporal motion tracking for deformable surfaces using stereo-video sequence is proposed. It is worth to highlight that none of these methods were designed to combine SfS and DSfM for elastic surface reconstruciton using one single view.

Contributions. The contribution of our work is three folds: *(i)* Combining SfS and DSfM, *(i)* reconstruction of a template albedo map of in-vivo human organs and *(iii)* using shading cues to recover deformations in regions where feature correspondences are missing and using feature correspondences as boundary conditions to the reconstruction with shading.

3   Notation and Geometric Characterization of Smooth Surfaces

A smooth surface Γ can be parameterized by a $\mathcal{C}^2$-function $\Phi\colon \Omega \subset \mathbb{R}^2 \to \mathbb{R}^3$: $(u,v) \mapsto \mathbf{Q} = \left(\Phi_x(u,v)\ \Phi_y(u,v)\ \Phi_z(u,v)\right)^{\top}$. We do not make a distinction between the surface Γ and the mapping Φ unless needed. We call template the surface at rest. The Jacobian of Φ, denoted J_Φ, is given by: $\mathsf{J}_\Phi = \begin{pmatrix} \frac{\partial \Phi_x}{\partial u} & \frac{\partial \Phi_y}{\partial u} & \frac{\partial \Phi_z}{\partial u} \\ \frac{\partial \Phi_x}{\partial v} & \frac{\partial \Phi_y}{\partial v} & \frac{\partial \Phi_z}{\partial v} \end{pmatrix}^{\top}$ It is a (3×2) matrix which at each $(u,v) \in \Omega$ maps a local unit square of Ω to a tangent plane at

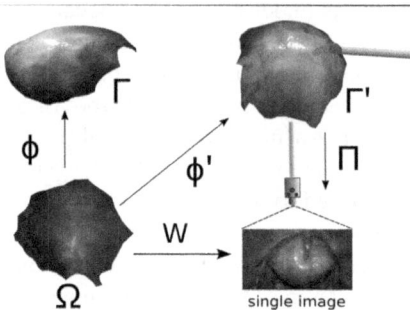

Fig. 2. Surface representation. Left: Φ is a conformal map. Geodesics on Ω, which is a flattening of Γ, are stretched on Γ. The angles tend to be preserved by Φ and area changes are tolerated. Φ' is the conformal map which reconstruct a deformation of the template Γ by the surgery tool. $\mathcal{W}$ is correspondence function between the template and the deformed image. In our work, Φ is computed during the exploration phase. $\mathcal{W}$ is computed from feature correspondences. Π is the projection matrix of a 3D point to the image plan including camera's intrinsics and Φ' is the unknown deformation function.

$\Phi(u, v)$. The normal of the surface at a point (u, v) is given by $\mathsf{N} = \left(\frac{\partial \Phi_x}{\partial u} \ \frac{\partial \Phi_y}{\partial u} \ \frac{\partial \Phi_z}{\partial u} \right)^{\top} \times \left(\frac{\partial \Phi_x}{\partial v} \ \frac{\partial \Phi_y}{\partial v} \ \frac{\partial \Phi_z}{\partial v} \right)^{\top}$. Where $\times$ stands for the cross product in $\mathbb{R}^3$. Let $\mathcal{W} \colon \Omega \to \mathbb{R}^2$ be a known warp which maps points from the template to surface points in the deformed image. The deformed image contains the projection of the deformed surface. In practice, $\mathcal{W}$ can be a function which matches features in the template and in the deformed image. Let $\Pi \colon \mathbb{R}^3 \to \mathbb{R}^2 \colon (x\,y\,z)^{\top} \mapsto (a\,b)^{\top}$ be the projection of a 3D point to the image plan.

4   Reconstruction of the Template's 3D Shape

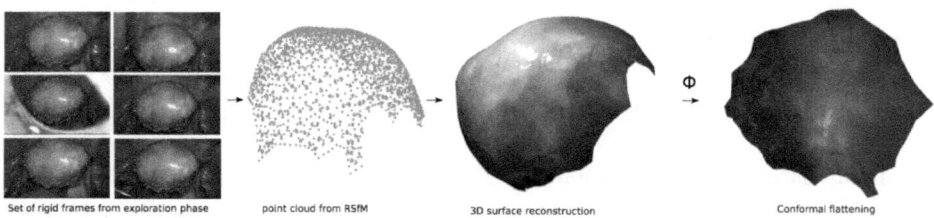

Fig. 3. Uterus template reconstruction during the exploration phase using a classic technique of Rigid SfM. From left-to-right: The rigid frames are combined to extract a dense point cloud of the uterus surface. Then, the 3D points are meshed and texture mapped. Finally, conformal flattening is applied.

As in [7], we assume that during the exploration of the peritoneal environment, the organs are at rest and the acquired image sequence undergoes a rigid motion of a rigid scene. This allows us to reconstruct both the template's 3D shape. From M views, Rigid SfM finds camera parameters as well as a set of 3D points $(x_j\ y_j\ z_j)$, $j = 1, \ldots, N_v$ which will be the template points. There are several ways to proceed for Rigid SfM [4]. We chose the classical sequential approach where two different views with enough baseline are used to compute the essential matrix, from which the relative camera position can be extracted and used to triangulate a first set of 3D points. The camera position, $\mathsf{T}_i, i = 1, \ldots, M - 1$, for each other view is then computed on turn using camera resection, and new 3D points are triangulated. Finally, bundle adjustment is launched to minimize the reprojection error, and the 3D points are connected to form a mesh with N_F faces $\mathcal{F}$ and N_v vertices $\mathcal{V}$ given by the set of triangulated 3D points. Image consistent meshing can be used [9]. Conformal flattening can be used to estimate the geometric parameterization of the obtained surface. The results of applying this method to an in-vivo video sequence from laparosurgery is shown in figure 3.

5   Reconstruction of the Template's Albedo

Several methods were proposed to estimate the albedo of a surface [11,20]. In the context of laparosurgery, the light source is rigidly mounted on the tip of the endoscope and then can be assumed as being co-linear to the axis of the camera's principal axis $\mathsf{L} = \begin{pmatrix} 0\ 0\ 1 \end{pmatrix}^{\top}$ (see figure 4). Assuming a Lambertian diffuse surface, the reflectance model expresses the image intensity at a pixel $\mathcal{W}(u, v)$ with respect to the surface normal $\mathsf{N}(u, v)$ and the direction of the distant light source L: $\mathcal{I}(\mathcal{W}(u, v)) = \alpha(u, v)\mathsf{L}\cot\mathsf{N}(u, v)$, with $\alpha(u, v)$ is the albedo of the surface. Using the reconstructed template 3D surface the normals $\mathsf{N}(u, v)$ can be easily computed. Given an image i, $i = 1, \ldots, M$, the corresponding albedo map can be estimated as:

$$\alpha_i(u, v) = \frac{\mathcal{I}_i(u, v)}{\mathsf{L} \cdot (\mathsf{R}_i\mathsf{N}(u, v))}, \quad i = 1, \ldots, M \tag{1}$$

where R_i is the rotation part of T_i. This equation is not defined when L is perpendicular to $\mathsf{R}_i\mathsf{N}(u, v)$. This situation can be easily detected since both vectors are known and $\alpha_i(u, v)$ is set to a pre-defined maximum value. Another interesting situation is when the light source direction is parallel to the surface normal and then the full projected light is reflected by the surface toward the camera. Usually this effect saturates the camera sensor and the corresponding area appears as specular shining white in the image. We finally define the albedo map by computing the minimum value at each pixel over all frames. This process handles specularities and most of the other unmodeled effects:

$$\alpha(u, v) = \min_{i\in\{1,\ldots,M\}} \alpha_i(u, v) \tag{2}$$

The obtained template's albedo of the in-vivo uterus sequence is displayed in figure 4.

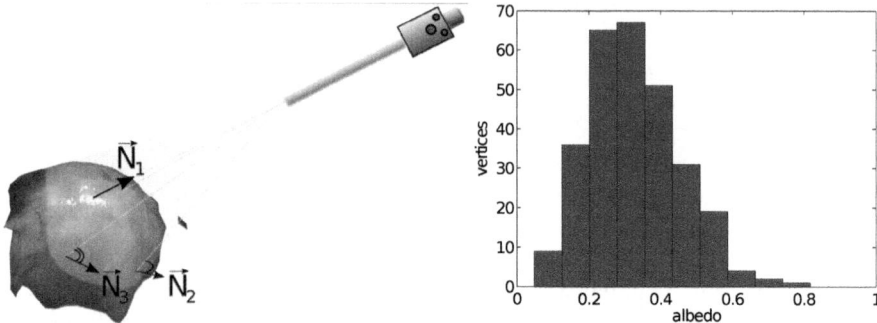

Fig. 4. Left: The image intensity at a surface point depends on the laparoscope's light source direction and the surface normal at that point. Points which have a normal parallel to the light direction produce specularities in the resulting image. Right: The histogram values of the albedo of the vertices.

6   Monocular Conformal Reconstruction

In [7] a discrete conformal reconstruction of deformable surfaces is proposed from N_c point correspondences between the deformed shape in an image and the 3D template $\Phi(u_i, v_i) \leftrightarrow \mathcal{W}(u_i, v_i)$, $i = 1, \ldots, N_c$. In the template, the correspondences are given by their barycentric coordinates $(f_i \; \mathsf{b}_i)^\top$, $i = 1, \ldots, N_c$, relatively to the triangle they lie on. In the image, the correspondences are given in pixel coordinates $\mathcal{W}(u_i, \; v_i)^\top$, $i = 1, \ldots, N_c$. Extensible 3D reconstruction was formulated in [7] as:

$$\min_{\mathcal{V}'} \sum_{i=1}^{N_c} \| \; \Pi(\mathsf{K} \; \mathsf{v}'(f_i) \mathsf{b}_i) - \mathcal{W}(u_i, v_i) \; \| \qquad \text{(motion)}$$
$$+\lambda_1 \sum_{i=1}^{N_F} \| \; \mathsf{S}_i - \mathsf{S}_i^0 \; \|^2 \qquad\qquad\qquad \text{(shearing)}$$
$$+\lambda_2 \sum_{i=1}^{N_F} \| \; \mathsf{A}_i - \mathsf{A}_i^0 \; \|^2 \qquad\qquad\qquad \text{(anisotropy)} \qquad (3)$$
$$+\lambda_3 \| \; \Delta \mathcal{V}' \; \|^2 \qquad\qquad\qquad\qquad \text{(smoothing)}$$

where K is the (3×3) intrinsic matrix of the camera, $\mathsf{v}'(f_i)$ is the (3×3) matrix whose columns are the 3D coordinates of the vertices of face i, S_i and A_i are the 2D shearing and anisotropy scaling transforms from the template to the deformed i^{th} face, λ_1 and λ_2 are two real positive weights that tune the importance of the shearing, the anisotropy scaling and the smoothing energy term. The combination of these two non-isometric transforms relaxes the inextensible condition and allows one to deal with local extensible deformations. S^0 and A^0 are average amounts of shearing and anisotropy for each face of the 3D template mesh. They can be either learned from training data or experimentally set. Practically, normalized shearing and anisotropy transforms are experimentally set and then scaled by the triangle area of each face f_i to obtain the transforms S_i^0 and A_i^0. The additional weighted energy term smoothes the deformed shape. It is expressed through the linear Laplace-Beltrami discrete linear operator Δ of dimension $N_v \times N_v$ [21]. $\mathcal{V}'$ is an $N_v \times 3$ matrix which concatenates the 3D mesh vertices $\mathcal{V}'_i$ of the reconstructed deformed mesh. This result is used as input to our monocular DSfMS method.

7 Monocular Conformal DSfMS

The resulting deformed shape with the set of vertices $\mathcal{V}_i'$, $i = 1, \ldots, N_v$, recovered from the previously described method can be refined using shading cues. Using the reconstructed template albedo values $\alpha(u_i, v_i)$, $i = 1, \ldots, N_v$ for each vertex, we formulate the conformal reconstruction with motion and shading cues reconstruction as:

$$\min_{\mathcal{V}''} \sum_{i=1}^{N_c} \left\| (0\ 0\ 1)^\top \mathbf{v}''(f_i) \begin{pmatrix} b_{1i} \\ b_{2i} \\ b_{3i} \end{pmatrix} - (0\ 0\ 1)^\top \mathbf{v}'(f_i) \begin{pmatrix} b_{1i} \\ b_{2i} \\ b_{3i} \end{pmatrix} \right\| + \quad \text{(boundary cond.)}$$

$$\lambda_4 \sum_{\substack{v \\ i=1}}^{N} \| \Pi(\mathsf{K}\mathbf{v}_i'') - \Pi(\mathsf{K}\mathbf{v}_i') \|^2 + \qquad\qquad\qquad \text{(reprojection cond.)}$$

$$\lambda_5 \sum_{i \in \mathcal{D}_v} \| \mathcal{I}'(\mathcal{W}''(u_i, v_i)) - \alpha(u_i, v_i)\mathsf{L}.\mathsf{N}''(u_i, v_i) \|^2 + \qquad \text{(diffuse vertices)}$$

$$\lambda_6 \sum_{i \in \mathcal{S}_v} \| \mathsf{L} \times \mathsf{N}''(u_i, v_i) \|^2 + \qquad\qquad\qquad\quad \text{(specular vertices)}$$

$$\lambda_7 \| \Delta \mathcal{V}'' \|^2 \qquad\qquad\qquad\qquad\qquad\qquad\qquad\quad \text{(smoothing)}$$

$$\tag{4}$$

where $\mathcal{D}_v$ and $\mathcal{S}_v$ are respectively the diffuse and specular vertices. The specular vertices can be easily detected as saturated regions in the deformed image intensity $\mathcal{I}'$. The real parameters $\lambda_4, \lambda_5, \lambda_6, \lambda_7$ are experimentally set. Through the boundary condition, this formulation gives confidence to the depth of the correspondences reconstructed by the conformal method using motion. The reprojection condition limits the refinement of the vertices along the camera sightlines. The diffuse condition refines the diffuse vertices according to the Lambertian model using shading. The specular vertices are constrained to have their normals parallel to the direction of the source light. Due to noise in the image intensity a smoothing term is needed to avoid bumpy surface reconstructions. The diffuse and specular terms allows us to recover the deformed surface in regions where the data correspondences are missing.

8 Experimental Results

8.1 Synthetic Data

The synthetic deformation model. The obtained template mesh is deformed to evaluate the performance of our approach with different amounts of edge extension and curvature changes. The synthetic deformation model enables us to simulate a push and pull by the surgeon's tool upon the uterus tissue. It is defined as a set of pairs of unit vectors $\mathbf{F}_j$ and attraction points $\mathbf{g}_j$: $\{(\mathbf{F}_j, \mathbf{g}_j)\}_{j \in J}$, $J = \{1, \ldots, d\}$. $\mathbf{F}_j$ represents the main direction of deformation toward the attraction point $\mathbf{g}_j$ and d is the number of attraction points. Given a pair $(\mathbf{F}_j, \mathbf{g}_j)$, the new location of a vertex of the template mesh is computed as: $\overrightarrow{\mathbf{v}_i \mathbf{v}_i'} = k((\mathbf{F}_j, \overrightarrow{\mathbf{v}_i \mathbf{g}_j})) \overrightarrow{\mathbf{v}_i \mathbf{g}_j} + \epsilon \mathbf{N}_i$, where $\mathbf{N}_i$ is the unit normal of the surface at the point $\mathbf{v}_i$, ϵ is a real number of small value used to move the vertex according to the tangent plan and avoid to drag it abruptly toward the attraction point. k is a function which models the effect of the attraction between $\mathbf{g}_j$ and $\mathbf{v}_i$. It is assumed to be dependent only on the angle between the main direction of deformation and the vector joining the vertex to the attraction point. The smaller this angle the bigger the effect of the attraction point on the vertex.

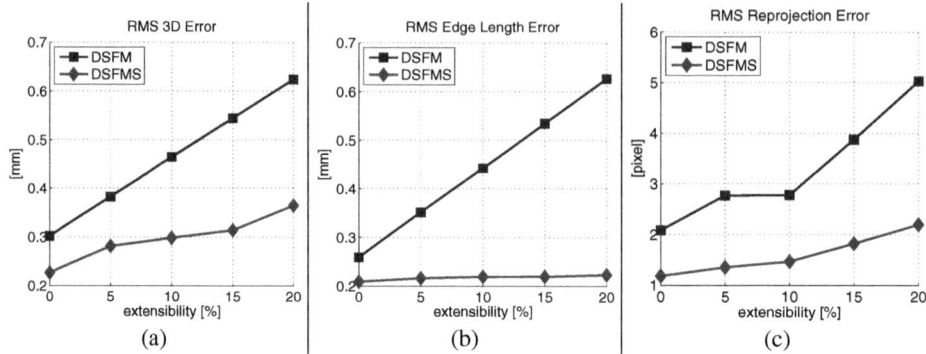

Fig. 5. 3D reconstruction error versus extensibility for conformal DSfM and DSfMS methods using the synthetic sequence *ext*

Results. A sequence of 500 deformations is produced so that the amount of extensibility *w.r.t.* the template varies as: $ext = [0\%\ 5\%\ 10\%\ 15\%\ 20\%]$. The deformed images are obtained by projecting each 3D deformed mesh using a perspective projection matrix Π. The intrinsics of this projection are taken as being the same as a Karl Storz laparoscope's intrinsics. A z-buffer rendering method is used to compute the self-occluded areas and to texture map the projected mesh. The point correspondences are from the 3D template mesh to 2D deformed image. They are obtained by randomly choosing 500 points represented by their barycentric coordinates. In the deformed mesh the points, which have the same barycentric coordinates, are projected using the same perspective projection matrix Π to obtain the 2D correspondences in the deformed image. We proceed to the evaluation of the developed method by adding Gaussian noise of zero mean and different variances to the 2D correspondences. Since in real in-vivo video sequence it is very difficult to automatically obtain correspondences in the deformed area due to the presence of the surgery tool and moving specularities, we do not consider any synthetic correspondences in the deformed area. Only 25 point correspondences are used between the 3D template and the 2D single input image. For lack of space, the qualitative reconstructed surface are not shown for DSfM and DSfMS. The quantitative results show the RMS 3D error of vertices is computed as the summed norm of the difference between reconstructed and ground truth vertices. The RMS edge length error is computed as the summed norm of difference of the mesh edge's lengths between reconstructed and ground truth surface. The reprojection error is computed as the summed norm of difference between the projection of the points in the reconstructed mesh and the corresponding in the deformed image. As expected, in the case of sparse feature correspondences, the DSfMS outperforms the DSfM method. When the number of correspondences is augmented in the deformed regions, the DSfM method tends to be as accurate as the proposed method.

8.2   Real Data

To validate the proposed approach on real data, the experiment we propose is the 3D reconstruction of an uterus from in-vivo sequences acquired using a monocular Karl

Storz laparoscope. The 3D template of the uterus is generated during the laparosurgery exploration step of the inside body. Then, a set of complex and unpredictible deformations may occur on the uterus when the surgeon starts to examine it. A set of 35 correspondences between the 3D uterus template and the deformed images was generated. The correspondences in deformed regions are either absent or non-stable and then are not taken into account. As it is hard to provide ground truth data to compare with, besides the quantitative results from the synthetic data, the qualitative 3D reconstruction shows clear improvement of the recovery of the deformed region with no need of point correspondences. Table 1 compares 3D reconstructed deformation with SfS, DSfM and the proposed DSfMS. As expected, the SfS method provide bumpy reconstructed surface due to specularities and unmodeled physical phenomena. The DSfM method provides coarse reconstruction since feature correspondences are missing in the deformed regions. DSfMS provides a finer and meaningful 3D reconstruction.

Table 1. 3D reconstruction on in-vivo video sequence from monocular laparoscope using SfS, DSfM and the proposed DSfMS. First row: Single 2D views of uterus deformation with a surgery tool. Second row: 3D reconstruction using SfS. Each 3D reconstruction is done using the single view above. The view is given in the laparoscope view point. Third row: 3D deformed surface seen from different point of view which provide visualization of the self-occluded part. Fourth row: Zoom in the deformed reconstructed area with DSfMS.

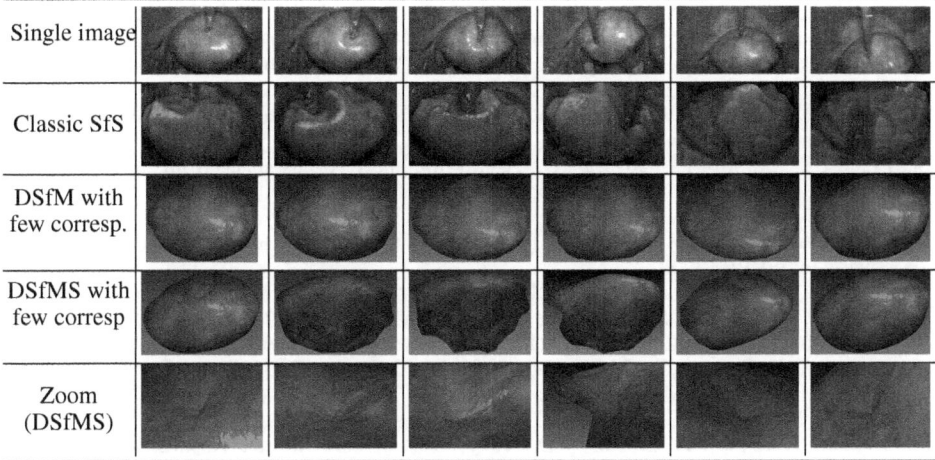

Single image					
Classic SfS					
DSfM with few corresp.					
DSfMS with few corresp					
Zoom (DSfMS)					

9 Conclusion

In this paper, we have presented the DSfMS method to reconstruct a conformal deforming living tissue in 3D by combining motion and shading cues. Our method provides novel technical contributions and also a new way of tackling the 3D vision problem in laparoscopy. The synthetic data and in-vivo experimental results show the ability of the proposed method to recover a smooth surface subjected to deformation in local region without correspondences.

References

1. Brunet, F., Hartley, R., Bartoli, A., Navab, N., Malgouyres, R.: Monocular Template-Based Reconstruction of Smooth and Inextensible Surfaces. In: Kimmel, R., Klette, R., Sugimoto, A. (eds.) ACCV 2010, Part III. LNCS, vol. 6494, pp. 52–66. Springer, Heidelberg (2011)
2. Grasa, O.G., Civera, J., Montiel, J.: EKF monocular slam with relocalization for laparoscopic sequences. In: ICRA (2011)
3. Hager, G., Vagvolgyi, B., Yuh, D.: Stereoscopic video overlay with deformable registration. Medicine Meets Virtual Reality (2007)
4. Hartley, R.I., Zisserman, A.: Multiple View Geometry in Computer Vision, 2nd edn. Cambridge University Press (2003)
5. Hayashibe, M., Suzuki, N., Hattori, A., Nakamura, Y.: Intraoperative Fast 3D Shape Recovery of Abdominal Organs in Laparoscopy. In: Dohi, T., Kikinis, R. (eds.) MICCAI 2002. LNCS, vol. 2489, pp. 356–363. Springer, Heidelberg (2002)
6. Hayashibe, M., Suzuki, N., Nakamura, Y.: Laser-scan endoscope system for intraoperativegeometry acquisition and surgical robot safety management. MIA 10, 509–519 (2006)
7. Malti, A., Bartoli, A., Collins, T.: Template-based conformal shape-from-motion from registered laparoscopic images. In: MIUA (2011)
8. Moreno-Noguer, F., Salzmann, M., Lepetit, V., Fua, P.: Capturing 3D stretchable surfaces from single images in closed form. In: CVPR (2009)
9. Morris, D.D., Kanade, T.: Image-consistent surface triangulation. In: CVPR (2000)
10. Nicolau, S.A., Pennec, X., Soler, L., Ayache, N.: A Complete Augmented Reality Guidance System for Liver Punctures: First Clinical Evaluation. In: Duncan, J.S., Gerig, G. (eds.) MICCAI 2005. LNCS, vol. 3749, pp. 539–547. Springer, Heidelberg (2005)
11. Nishino, K., Zhang, Z., Ikeuchi, K.: Illumination distribution from a sparse set of images for view-dependent image synthesis. In: ICCV (2001)
12. Penne, J., Höller, K., Stürmer, M., Schrauder, T., Schneider, A., Engelbrecht, R., Feußner, H., Schmauss, B., Hornegger, J.: Time-of-Flight 3-D Endoscopy. In: Yang, G.-Z., Hawkes, D., Rueckert, D., Noble, A., Taylor, C. (eds.) MICCAI 2009. LNCS, vol. 5761, pp. 467–474. Springer, Heidelberg (2009)
13. Perriollat, M., Hartley, R., Bartoli, A.: Monocular template-based reconstruction of inextensible surfaces. In: BMVC (2008)
14. Prados, E., Camilli, F., Faugeras, O.: A unifying and rigorous shape from shading method adapted to realistic data and applications. Journal of Mathematical Imaging and Vision 25(3), 307–328 (2006)
15. Salzmann, M., Urtasun, R., Fua, P.: Local deformation models for monocular 3D shape recovery. In: CVPR (2008)
16. Stoyanov, D., Darzi, A., Yang, G.Z.: Dense 3D Depth Recovery for Soft Tissue Deformation During Robotically Assisted Laparoscopic Surgery. In: Barillot, C., Haynor, D.R., Hellier, P. (eds.) MICCAI 2004. LNCS, vol. 3217, pp. 41–48. Springer, Heidelberg (2004)
17. Stoyanov, D., Scarzanella, M.V., Pratt, P., Yang, G.-Z.: Real-Time Stereo Reconstruction in Robotically Assisted Minimally Invasive Surgery. In: Jiang, T., et al. (eds.) MICCAI 2010, Part I. LNCS, vol. 6361, pp. 275–282. Springer, Heidelberg (2010)
18. Totz, J., Mountney, P., Stoyanov, D., Yang, G.-Z.: Dense Surface Reconstruction for Enhanced Navigation in MIS. In: Fichtinger, G., Martel, A., Peters, T. (eds.) MICCAI 2011, Part I. LNCS, vol. 6891, pp. 89–96. Springer, Heidelberg (2011)
19. Winter, M.: Image-Based Incremental Reconstruction, Rendering and Augmented Visualziation of Surfaces for Endoscopic Surgery. PhD thesis, University of Erlangen (2009)
20. Wu, C., Varanasi, K., Liu, Y., Seidel, H.-P., Theobalt, C.: Shading-based dynamic shape refinement from multi-view video under general illumination. In: ICCV (2011)
21. Yoo, D.: Three-dimensional morphing of similar shapes using a template mesh. International Journal of Precision Engineering and Manufacturing (2009)
22. Zhang, L., Curless, B., Hertzmann, A., Seitz, S.M.: Shape and motion under varying illumination: Unifying structure from motion, photometric stereo, and multi-view stereo. In: ICCV (2003)
23. Zhang, R., Tsai, P.-S., Cryer, J.E., Shah, M.: Shape from shading: A survey. PAMI 21(8), 690–706 (1999)

Towards Live Monocular 3D Laparoscopy Using Shading and Specularity Information

Toby Collins and Adrien Bartoli

ALCoV-ISIT
Université d'Auvergne, Clermont-Ferrand, France
{Toby.Collins,Adrien.Bartoli}@gmail.com

Abstract. We present steps toward the first real-time system for computing and visualising 3D surfaces viewed in live monocular laparoscopy video. Our method is based on estimating 3D shape using shading and specularity information, and seeks to push current Shape from Shading (SfS) boundaries towards practical, reliable reconstruction. We present an accurate method to model any laparoscope's light source, and a highly-parallelised SfS algorithm that outperforms the fastest current method. We give details of its GPU implementation that facilitates realtime performance of an average frame-rate of 23fps. Our system also incorporates live 3D visualisation with virtual stereoscopic synthesis. We have evaluated using real laparoscopic data with ground-truth, and we present the successful in-vivo reconstruction of the human uterus. We however draw the conclusion that the shading cue alone is insufficient to reliably handle arbitrary laparoscopic images.

1 Introduction

An important computer vision task in Minimally Invasive Surgery (MIS) is to recover the 3D structure of organs and tissues viewed in laparoscopic images and videos. A general solution to this has important applications, including depth estimation and perception, enhanced intra-operative surgical guidance, motion estimation and compensation, pre-operative data registration and novel-view synthesis. Currently, state-of-the-art methods for acquiring 3D information differ along two main axes; (i) the sensor hardware used to estimate 3D, and (ii) the visual cue used to infer 3D shape. 3D reconstruction has been attempted previously by modifying traditional monocular laparoscopes; these include stereo laparoscopes [14,4] and active 3D methods based on structured light [1] and Time-of-Flight cameras [12]. These simplify the reconstruction problem, yet come at the price of additional intra-operative hardware. Furthermore, these have not been shown to work with a great degree of accuracy in practice. Stereo laparoscopes can also be used purely for 3D visualisation. However, resolving the difference between the camera's convergence angles and the user's eyes prove to be the limitation [8]. By contrast, monocular methods require no hardware modification and aim to estimate 3D shape from 2D data. Virtual stereo images can easily be visualised which match the convergence angle of the user's eyes.

P. Abolmaesumi et al. (Eds.): IPCAI 2012, LNAI 7330, pp. 11–21, 2012.
© Springer-Verlag Berlin Heidelberg 2012

However, the 3D reconstruction problem is considerably more difficult, and remains an open challenge. Shape from Motion (SfM) is one monocular method gaining some ground. The most successful are based on realtime Simultaneous Localisation And Mapping (SLAM) [7,3]. However, these require correspondence estimation; a very difficult task in laparoscopic images. Also SLAM assumes the 3D scene is either rigid or adheres to a very strict motion model, which is mostly unrealistic during intervention. Shape from Shading (SfS) is another monocular method based on the relationship between 3D geometry, surface reflectance and scene illumination. It is a strong contender for monocular 3D laparoscopy since it (*i*) requires no correspondence, (*ii*) requires only a single input image and (*iii*) in laparoscopy the light conditions are highly controlled.However, SfS is a *weakly constrained problem*, and real conditions in laparoscopy often violate its core assumptions. Our overarching research goal is to answer the following two questions: *1. Is SfS a viable method for monocular 3D laparoscopy? 2. Is SfS sufficient on its own, or must it be complemented by other 3D cues?* In parallel to answering these questions, we have been developing a live (i.e. realtime) SfS-based 3D reconstruction/visualisation system (Fig. 1).

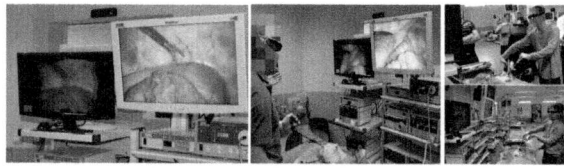

Fig. 1. Our current live monocular 3D laparoscopy prototype system. (Left): Two screens showing (white) the raw 2D video feed and (black) the reconstructed 3D with an active-shutter display. (Remaining images): System in use.

In this paper we extend the boundaries of SfS by improving some of the various modelling and computation aspects. We present a new way to accurately model a laparoscopic light source with what we call the *Nonparametric Light Model* (NLM). We show how to calibrate this easily and how it is incorporated into SfS. We also present a highly-parallelised shape estimation algorithm, which facilitates realtime 3D reconstruction. What we do not do is claim to have solved SfS for laparoscopy. There exist several open modelling, optimisation and practical challenges not addressed. We clearly state these in §1.2, to help guide other researches towards completing the problem.

1.1   Problem Statement

We briefly describe here the SfS image irradiance equation, which is the basis for all SfS methods. We then summarise its various instantiations from the state-of-the-art. Let us define a 3D surface S that is parameterized by the function $f(u,v) : \mathbb{R}^2 \to \mathbb{R}^3$. This maps some point (u,v) on the surface's domain into the camera's 3D coordinate frame. The Lambertian model predicts the *image irradiance* (the amount of light hitting the camera's CCD) according to:

$$g(\hat{I}\,(\psi(f(u,v)))) = \alpha(u,v)\mathcal{L}(f\,(u,v)) \cdot n(u,v) + \varepsilon \qquad (1)$$

Here, the function $g : \mathbb{R} \to \mathbb{R}$ denotes the camera's response function, which coverts pixel intensities into image irradiance. $\psi\,(f\,(u,v)) = (x,y)$ denotes the 3D-to-2D camera projection process. $\hat{I}\,(x,y)$ denotes the measured pixel intensity at pixel (x,y). $\alpha\,(u,v)$ denotes the surface albedo and $n\,(u,v)$ denotes the surface normal. ε denotes pixel measurement noise. The illumination vector $\mathcal{L}\,(f\,(u,v)) = [l_x, l_y, l_z] : \mathbb{R}^3 \to \mathbb{R}^3$ models the illumination as a directed ray of light. In classic SfS (u,v) spans a closed region in the input image: $\Omega \in \mathbb{R}^2$. The surface function $f\,(u,v)$ is then determined by the *depth function* $d\,(u,v) : \mathbb{R}^3 \to \mathbb{R}$. For perspective cameras, this is given by $f\,(u,v) = d\,(u,v)\,\mathbf{K}^{-1}\,(u,v,1)^\top$, where $\mathbf{K}$ is the matrix of camera intrinsics. The goal of SfS is to estimate $d\,(u,v)$ given intensity measurements at each pixel using (1). This is given by:

$$d^\star\,(u,v) = \arg\min_{d(u,v)} \int_{\Omega} (\alpha\,(u,v)\,\mathcal{L}\,(f\,(u,v)) \cdot n\,(u,v) - g(\hat{I}\,(u,v)))^2 du dv \qquad (2)$$

1.2 Solving SfS: State-Of-The-Art

All SfS methods attempt to solve Problem (2), yet this is a highly non-trivial, often ill-posed problem. The specifics of an SfS method can be broken into three key components. These are: (*i*) **Modelling** the image formation process, (*ii*) making **scene assumptions** about the 3D environment and (*iii*) **3D computation** via optimisation. In Fig. (2) we present these three key SfS components. The table's second row summarises how they have been instantiated by recent works. In this paper we attempt to push forward the boundaries of SfS for 3D laparoscopy, but which permit effective realtime optimisation. Our core contributions are represented clearly in green.

	Modelling				Scene Assumptions		3D Computation	
	Camera Response Model	Illumination Model	Reflectance Model	Projection Model	Surface Albedo	Surface Discontinuities	Processing Time	Optimality
State Of The Art	Known & Constant	PLM & Constant	Lambertian	Perspective & Constant	Known & Constant	No Discontinuities	Not realtime*	Local&Global
Proposed Developments	Known & Constant	Accurate & Constant	Lambertian & specularities	Perspective & Constant	Small Improvement	No Discontinuities	Realtime	Local

Fig. 2. The three key components of SfS. Second row: current state-of-the-art. Third row: Our proposed developments specifically for 3D laparoscopy.

State-of-the-art methods require the camera response function to be known. There are no methods which can simultaneously adjust the response function in a video and perform SfS. This however is needed if the camera's exposure or shutter speed changes. For the illumination source, the Point Light Model (PLM) has been proposed for endoscopes [11,18]. This uses the inverse-squared light falloff model. Regarding the reflectance model, all SfS methods applied to endoscopy have used Lambertian reflectance [13,19,18,15,9]. This makes the modelling problem less challenging, but is less accurate thane the the the full BRDF. Regarding the camera model, the perspective model was proposed in [10,16]. However, no existing method can handle unknown and changing camera intrinsics in a video, caused by zooming, for example. The scene assumptions in SfS nearly always involve fixed, constant and known surface albedo. Some recent progress towards piecewise-constant albedo has been proposed in [2] using learned natural image statistics. Since most SfS methods provide constraints on surface normals, they cannot handle discontinuous surfaces. Regarding the 3D computation, with the exception of Tsai and Shai (TS) [17] (noted by *), the SfS methods cannot run in realtime on today's hardware. However TS use models which are poor in laparoscopic conditions, such as an orthographic camera and Distant Light Model (DLM). SfS methods can also be broken into locally or globally-optimal [19] solutions. Global solutions are however slow to compute.

2   Accurately Modelling a Laparoscope's Light Source

In this section we present the Nonparametric Light Model (NLM). In contrast to the DLM and PLM, which are poor approximations to the laparoscope's light source, one in fact cannot do better than the NLM. This is because it can model light functions of arbitrary complexity. We are however motivated by practical considerations regarding easy calibration. We have developed a one-time, fully automatic method that requires only multiple views of a planar calibration target. We use the NLM to compute $\mathcal{L}$ as a spatially-varying function defined at every 3D point bound within the operational volume of the laparoscope. It uses the premise that the illumination can be *locally modelled* at any 3D point $\mathbf{p} = (x, y, z)^{\top}$ by a local proximal light source. That is, $\mathcal{L}(\mathbf{p}) = [l_x, l_y, l_z]$, with $[l_x, l_y, l_z]$ being a local light vector of power $\|l_x, l_y, l_z\|$ and direction $[l_x, l_y, l_z] / \|l_x, l_y, l_z\|$. This model generalises both the DLM and PLM. The advantage of the NLM is that it can model well any of the various laparoscope light sources. Fig. 3(a) shows two examples we have modelled.

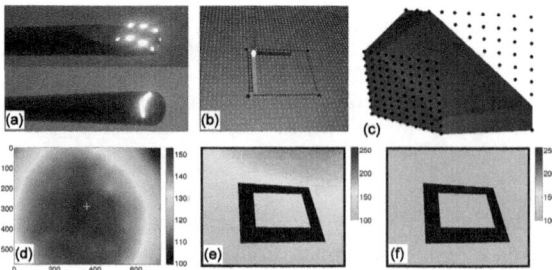

Fig. 3. Nonparametric Light Model: Calibration, modelling and accuracy

2.1   Calibrating the Nonparametric Light Model

To determine the function $\mathcal{L}$ the NLM must first be *calibrated*. We do this by using (1) and a ground-truth calibration object whose depths, normals and albedos are known. For convenience a planar calibration object is chosen with a tracking target printed on its surface. With this its 3D pose can be estimated robustly using well known methods [5] (Fig. 3(b)). Suppose the rigid transform $\mathbf{M} = [\mathbf{R}\,\mathbf{t}]$ maps the plane into the camera's coordinate frame. The surface function is then given by $f(u, v) = [\mathbf{R}_1\,\mathbf{R}_2]\,[u, v]^\top + \mathbf{t}$ and $n(u, v) = \mathbf{R}_3$, where $\mathbf{R}_i$ denotes the ith column of $\mathbf{R}$. Now that we have the surface function, at each pixel we obtain a sparse collection of linear constraints on $\mathcal{L}(\mathbf{p})$ according to (1). Our method for calibration involves recording a video of the plane as it moves through the laparoscope's operational 3D volume. At each frame, we accumulate constraints at slices of the volume, and over the video we acquire enough data to learn $\mathcal{L}$. Importantly, the plane must be recorded at multiple orientations (a minimum of 3). This is because there are three unknowns (l_x, l_y and l_z) at any given point.

In practice we can expect a finite number of noisy measurements. Denote these by the set $\{\hat{\mathbf{I}}_i, \mathbf{n}_i, \mathbf{p}_i\}$. However, to estimate the continuous function $\mathcal{L}$, a unique solution can be found using regularised function approximation. We propose using the 3D Thin Plate Spline (TPS) which has several desirable properties for us. It is globally smooth, easily computable, and contains the least possible nonlinear component to achieve the function approximation. The 3D TPS defines a set of n 3D control points that we position throughout the volume (Fig. 3(c) shows control points at the front and back planes of the 3D volume). The TPS model takes the form: $\mathcal{L}(\mathbf{p}) = \mathbf{a}(\mathbf{p})[\mathbf{S}^\top, \mathbf{1}]^\top$, where $\mathbf{a}(\mathbf{p})$ is a vector which depends locally on $\mathbf{p}$. The function is parameterised by an $n \times 3$ control matrix $\mathbf{S}$. Calibrating the NLM involves determining $\mathbf{S}$. We pose this as minimising the following quadratic least squares objective function:

$$\hat{\mathbf{S}} = \arg\min_{\mathbf{S}} \sum_i \left(\alpha_i \mathbf{a}_i [\mathbf{S}^\top, \mathbf{1}]^\top \mathbf{n}_i - g(\hat{I}_i) \right)^2 \tag{3}$$

Since $\mathbf{n}_i$ is expected to be noisy, we have a least squares problem with Errors In Variables. Thus we solve 3 using Total Least Squares. Once estimated, $\mathcal{L}(\mathbf{p})$ can be evaluated everywhere with $\mathcal{L}(x, y, z) = \mathbf{a}(\mathbf{p})[\hat{\mathbf{S}}^\top, \mathbf{1}]^\top$. Figs. 3(c,d) shows the NLM for the laparoscope in Figs. 3(a-bottom). A 1 minute video of the planar target was recorded (1,800 frames), whose depth ranged between 10mm to 110mm from the laparoscope tip. A TPS grid of $10 \times 10 \times 7$ was used to construct the NLM. Fig. 3(d) shows a cross-section of $\mathcal{L}$ at depth 15mm.

We can easily show the NLM is a far better model than the PLM. In Fig. 3(e) we show the predicted surface albedo, according to (1), for the plane in Fig. 3(b) assuming the PLM. The plane's true albedo is a constant $\alpha = 100$, but note that the albedo estimate towards the back is over double at the front, indicating a gross modelling error. By contrast, Fig. 3(f) shows a far better predicted albedo using the NLM. Note that this view was not used for training the model.

3   Parallelised 3D Depth Estimation

We return now to optimising (1), but now using our improved light model. For
realtime performance our solution is inspired by TS. We compute a discretised
version of (1), solved iteratively with depth estimates being updated fast, locally
and in parallel. However, our key extensions are (i) to handle perspective cameras, (ii) to handle general light models (including our NLM), (iii) guaranteeing
convergence and (iv computes smooth surfaces. We discretise (2) using the pixel
grid and augment it with a smoothing prior. This takes the form:

$$d^{\star}(u,v) = \underset{d(u,v)}{\arg\min}\sum_{\Omega}(\alpha(u,v)\,\mathcal{L}\,(f(u,v))\cdot n(u,v) - \hat{I}(u,v))^2\triangle u\triangle v +$$
$$\lambda\sum_{\Omega}\left(\tfrac{d}{du}f(u,v) + \tfrac{d}{dv}f(u,v)\right)^2 \quad (4)$$

λ denotes the smoothing term, which we currently experimentally set. At the
$(t+1)^{th}$ iteration the depth at (u,v) is updated by:

$$d^{t+1}(u,v) = \underset{d}{\arg\min}\left[\begin{array}{c}\left(\alpha(u,v)\,\mathcal{L}\,(f(u,v))\cdot n(u,v;d) - \hat{I}(u,v)\right)^2 + \\ \lambda\left(\tfrac{d}{du}f(u,v) + \tfrac{d}{dv}f(u,v)\right)\end{array}\right] \quad (5)$$

where the local surface normal $n(u,v;d)$ is computed by finite differences:

$$n(u,v;d) = \frac{1}{z(d)}\left[\begin{array}{c}\left(d\mathbf{K}^{-1}(u,v,1)^{\top} - d^t(u+1,v)\,\mathbf{K}^{-1}(u+1,v,1)^{\top}\right)\times \\ \left(d\mathbf{K}^{-1}(u,v,1)^{\top} - d^t(u+1,v)\,\mathbf{K}^{-1}(u+1,v,1)^{\top}\right)\end{array}\right] \quad (6)$$

Here, $z(d)$ denotes the normalisation term such that $\|n(u,v;d)\|_2 = 1$. To op-
timise efficiently, we sample candidate depths about the current depth estimate
in log-space via the rule: $d^{t+1}(u,v) \in \pm[d^t(u,v) + (1+\tau)^a - 1]$ with $\tau = 0.1$
and the integer a in the range: $a \in [0:10]$.

4   Algorithm and GPU Implementation

In this section we outline the details and some of the main design decisions we
have made in implementing live 3D laparoscopy using the methods described in
§2 and §3. Importantly, each input frame is processed independently, and thus
does not rely on the 3D computed in previous or successive frames.

4.1   Hardware Configuration and Offline Processing

Our current hardware configuration is as follows: A Karl Storz laparoscope with
video outputted via firewire at 720×576, a Windows 7 PC with an Intel Core2
Duo 3000MHz processor and NVidia Quadro FX 3800 card (with 192 CUDA
cores). For 3D visualisation we use a single Acer 25 Inch LCD 3D display combined with 4 pairs of NVidia 3D active shutter glasses. The laparoscope's automatic exposure is turned off (typically we set it to a 1/500 sec exposure) and
before running our reconstruction algorithm its camera is radiometrically and
geometrically calibrated. After calibrating the NLM, we precompute the function

$\mathcal{L}$ and store it as a $720 \times 576 \times 20$ quantised 3D frustum (requiring approximately 47MB of storage.) When processing live laparoscope videos, values from the NLM are then computed by 3D bilinear interpolation.

4.2 Online Processing

Input frames are captured from the laparoscope using the OpenCV libraries. We have found experimentally that the red channel best satisfies the constant albedo assumption for tissues in laparoscopy. We transfer the red channel to the GPU's DRAM. Subsequently all processing is done on the GPU. We report here the average absolute time to complete each process (in ms), and the process's percentage of the runtime budget.

Specular Constraints and Inpainting. (6.3ms, 14.2%) First, specularities are detected via combined saturation and lightness thresholding (we use thresholds of saturation 0.9 and lightness 0.95 respectively to detect specular pixels.) A rigorous modelling of specularities involves having physical reflectance models of tissue, which can be hard to apply in general. We opt for a simpler strategy: Our trick with processing specular pixels is to modify their intensity to that which would be predicted by Lambertian reflectance, and then running our SfS method. The process works by constraining each specular region's centroid to have maximal Lambertian reflectance. This is a reasonable estimate at its true Lambertian reflectance, because for a laparoscope the viewing rays and light rays are approximately colinear at these points. We then smoothly propagate this through the specular region.

Removal of High-Frequency Content. (2.8ms, 6.4%) We make the assumption that high frequency changes in image structure are caused by artifacts such as vascular structure, and not by shading variation. These are removed by running a GPU-optimised 7×7 media filter over the image.

Depth Map Initialisation and Estimation. (34.3ms, 77.3%) We initialise the depth map to be a fronto-parallel plane positioned at a 50mm from the laparoscope's end. We then run our SfS method until convergence is detected or if 30 iterations have passed. At each iteration, the pixel depths are updated in checkerboard fashion and in parallel on the GPU.

3D Visualisation. (0.93ms, 2.1%) Once the depth map has been estimated, we render two views of the 3D surface using stereoscopic OpenGL, and pass these to the FX 3800's quad buffers. Currently a parallel binocular setup is used, with cameras positioned either side of the real laparoscope camera model. Their parameters, including stereo baseline and 3D position are completely controllable.

5 Experimental Evaluation

5.1 Ex-vivo Experiments

To quanify the performance of our approach and to understand the general limitations of SfS for 3D laparoscopic reconstruction, we first present results

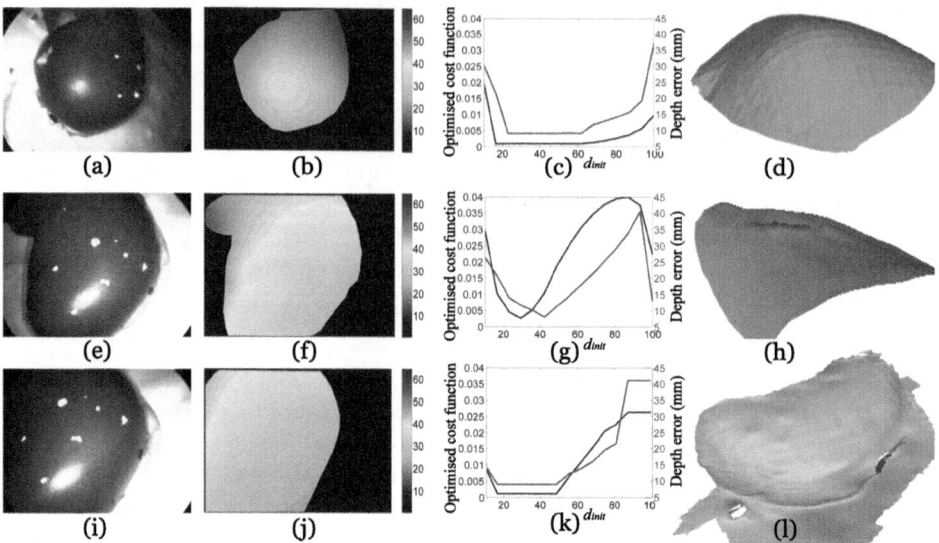

Fig. 4. Ex-vivo experimentation using a pig kidney with ground truth evaluation

for reconstructing ex-vivo a piglet's kidney. The analysis is presented in Figure 4. The kidney has been augmented with small white markers to provide the transform between the laparoscope's view and a Ground Truth (GT) surface, captured via a high-resolution structured light system (Fig. 4(l)). Three test laparoscope images are shown in Figs. 4 (a,e,i). Our goal here is to understand three key aspects: the well-posedness of the problem, the accuracy of the reconstruction and to measure the sensitivity of our approach to initialisation. We achieve this by manually segmenting the kidney and running the SfS method, initialised by fronto-parallel depth maps positioned at increasing depths d_{init}, ranging from 10mm < d_{init} < 100mm. Now, a well-posed problem is indicated by a unique global minima of the cost function (4). By contrast, the sensitivity to initialisation is indicated by measuring, for each value of d_{init}, the post-optimisation RMS Error w.r.t true depth. We illustrate the results graphically in Figs. 4(b,f,j). In Fig. 4(b) one can see the same (global) minima is reached between 20mm < d_{init} < 60mm mm, indicating reasonable resistance to coarse initialisation. The solutions for d_{init} > 60mm and d_{init} < 20mm have higher reconstruction error, however they also are marked by a higher cost function. This suggests that for image Fig. 4(a), the problem is well-posed. The reconstructed depth map for d_{init} = 50mm is shown in Fig. 4(c), and a 3D render of the visible surface from a novel viewpoint is shown in Fig. 4(d). For images in Figs. 4(e,i) we have similar results. However, the depth maps contain an error. At the bottom right of the kidney, the reconstructed depths tend closer to the camera, suggesting the surface here is concave. This is incorrect. Thus, there exists a convex/concave ambiguity and a non-unique solution. Returning back to the question posed in §1: *Is SfS sufficient to resolve 3D depth using monocular laparoscopes?* the answer in these images is not entirely, and another cue (such as motion) is needed to resolve the ambiguity.

5.2   Successful In-vivo Reconstruction

§5.1 shows reasonable 3D can be obtained via our SfS method, although failures can arise due to pose ambiguities. Here we show an in-vivo video sequence where 3D has been successfully reconstructed. The sequence is of a human uterus comprising 340 frames lasting 14.8 seconds [6]. We are specifically motivated by the application of computer-assisted myoma removal, where intra-operative 3D reconstruction can aid pre-operative data registration. This allows for example, visual augmentation of the fist planned incision path. The results on this dataset are summarised in Fig. 5. In Fig. 5(a-d) we show four representative frames from the sequence. In Figs. 5(e-g) we show the automatic image preprocessing done before running SfS. Fig. 5(e) is a raw input frame, Fig. 5(f) is the red channel after high-frequency content removal with detected specularities, Fig. 5(g) shows the image after specular inpainting. The uterus remains approximately rigid in the first half of the sequence. Our key idea is to evaluate our SfS method by constructing *in-vivo* quasi-GT 3D data using rigid SfM on these frames. To do this, a ROI was manually marked around the uterus (Fig. 5 (h)) and a dense GT surface bound by the ROI was computed using standard manually-assisted multiview SfM methods. We show this in Fig. 5(i). We processed the video sequence using two methods: (1) Tsai and Shah (TS) and (2) our proposed method. Note

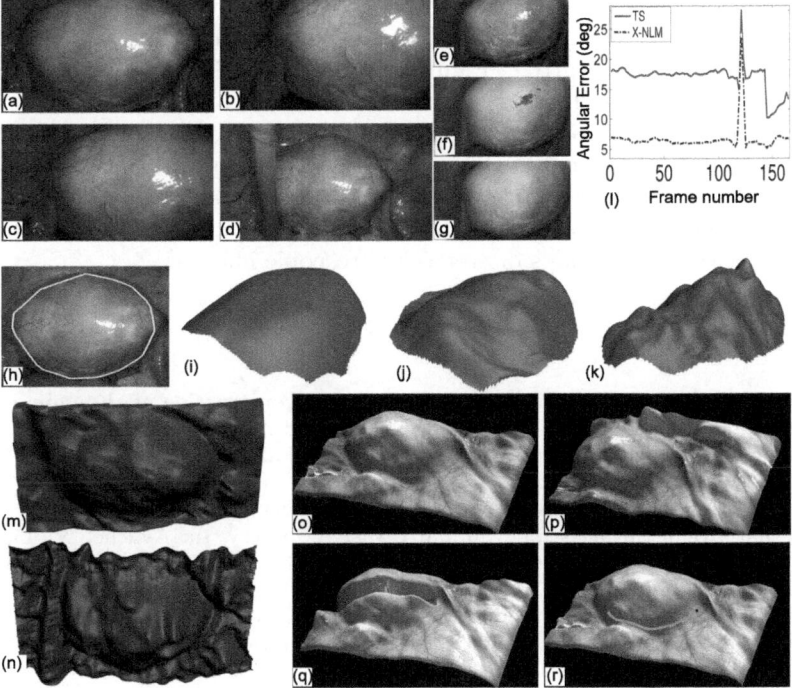

Fig. 5. Successful in-vivo 3D reconstruction of the human uterus

that in TS absolute depth cannot be computed. To enable quantative comparison, we compute the mean error in surface normals (in angular degrees). These scores are computed at each pixel bound within the visible part of the uterus.

Fig. 5(j) shows the reconstruction by our method for Fig. 5(h) and Fig. 5(k) shows it reconstructed by TS. Qualitatively, we ours appears superior to TS. In Fig. 5(l) we compare the reconstruction error of TS to ours (labelled as X-NLM). Here TS is noticeably outperformed by our method. The instrument occluded the uterus between frames 117-125, which explains the error spike. However, notices that since frames are processed independently, this has no adverse effect on successive frames. In Fig. 5(m,n) we show the full-image reconstruction using our method and TS respectively for the frame in Fig. 5(d). We note that no segmentation of the tool was performed, and the tissues surrounding the uterus violate the surface continuity and constant albedo assumptions. In spite of this, the uterus is recovered faithfully using our method. In Figs. 5(o,p,q) we show synthesised novel views, texture-mapped using the input image frames. In 5(q) the tool occludes the uterus, explaining the tool-shaped valley in the reconstruction. In Fig. 5(r) we show a basic application; we take 3D SfS surface and visually augment it with the pre-opetative planned incision path (shown in green).

6   Discussion and Conclusion

In this paper we have pushed forward SfS for live 3D monocular laparoscopy in various modelling and computational aspects. The contributions and outstanding weaknesses are stated clearly in Figure 2. The biggest limitations not addressed by our work are two-fold: (i): the surface albedo must be constant and known *a priori* and (ii) solution ambiguities due to the ill-conditioning of SfS. We believe they are tremendously difficult to resolve using the shading cue alone. Our direction for future research will be to take our live reconstruction framework and compliment it with other 3D cues. For example using sparse realtime 3D estimates at tracked features or stereo laparoscopic images.

References

1. Ackerman, J. D., Keller, K., Fuchs, H. Surface reconstruction of abdominal organs using laparoscopic structured light for augmented reality. 3DICA (2002)
2. Barron, J.T., Malik, J.: High-frequency shape and albedo from shading. In: CVPR, pp. 2521–2528 (2011)
3. Hu, M., Penney, G., Edwards, P., Figl, M., Hawkes, D.: 3D Reconstruction of Internal Organ Surfaces for Minimal Invasive Surgery. In: Ayache, N., Ourselin, S., Maeder, A. (eds.) MICCAI 2007, Part I. LNCS, vol. 4791, pp. 68–77. Springer, Heidelberg (2007)
4. Lau, W.W., Ramey, N.A., Corso, J.J., Thakor, N.V., Hager, G.D.: Stereo-Based Endoscopic Tracking of Cardiac Surface Deformation. In: Barillot, C., Haynor, D.R., Hellier, P. (eds.) MICCAI 2004. LNCS, vol. 3217, pp. 494–501. Springer, Heidelberg (2004)
5. Lepetit, V., Moreno-Noguer, F., Fua, P.: EPnP: An Accurate O(n) Solution to the PnP Problem. IJCV 81, 155–166 (2008)

6. Malti, A., Bartoli, A., Collins, T.: Template-Based Conformal Shape-from-Motion from Registered Laparoscopic Images. In: MIUA (2011)
7. Mountney, P., Yang, G.-Z.: Motion Compensated SLAM for Image Guided Surgery. In: Jiang, T., Navab, N., Pluim, J.P.W., Viergever, M.A. (eds.) MICCAI 2010. LNCS, vol. 6362, pp. 496–504. Springer, Heidelberg (2010)
8. Mueller-Richter, U.D.A., Limberger, A., Weber, P., Ruprecht, K.W., Spitzer, W., Schilling, M.: Possibilities and limitations of current stereo-endoscopy. Surgical Endoscopy 18, 942–947 (2004)
9. Okatani, T., Deguchi, K.: Shape reconstruction from an endoscope image by shape from shading technique for a point light source at the projection center. CVIU 66, 119–131 (1997)
10. Prados, E., Faugeras, O.: Perspective Shape from Shading and Viscosity Solutions. In: ICCV, pp. 826–831 (2003)
11. Prados, E., Faugeras, O.: Shape from Shading: a well-posed problem? In: CVPR, pp. 870–877 (2005)
12. Penne, J., Höller, K., Stürmer, M., Schrauder, T., Schneider, A., Engelbrecht, R., Feußner, H., Schmauss, B., Hornegger, J.: Time-of-Flight 3-D Endoscopy. In: Yang, G.-Z., Hawkes, D., Rueckert, D., Noble, A., Taylor, C. (eds.) MICCAI 2009. LNCS, vol. 5761, pp. 467–474. Springer, Heidelberg (2009)
13. Quartucci, C.H., Tozzi, C.L.: Towards 3D Reconstruction of Endoscope Images using Shape from Shading. In: SIBGRAPI, pp. 90–96 (2000)
14. Stoyanov, D., Darzi, A., Yang, G.Z.: Dense 3D Depth Recovery for Soft Tissue Deformation During Robotically Assisted Laparoscopic Surgery. In: Barillot, C., Haynor, D.R., Hellier, P. (eds.) MICCAI 2004. LNCS, vol. 3217, pp. 41–48. Springer, Heidelberg (2004)
15. Tankus, A., Sochen, N., Yeshurun, Y.: Perspective SfS by fast marching. In: CVPR, pp. 43–49 (2004)
16. Tankus, A., Sochen, N., Yeshurun, Y.: Shape-from-Shading Under Perspective Projection. IJCV 63, 21–43 (2007)
17. Tsai, P., Shah, M.: Shape From Shading Using Linear Approximation. Image and Vision Computing 12, 487–498 (1994)
18. Wu, C., Narasimhan, S.G., Jaramaz, B.: Shape-from-Shading under Near Point Lighting and Partial views for Orthopedic Endoscopy. In: PACV (2007)
19. Yeung, S.Y., Tsui, H.T., Yim, A.: Global Shape from Shading for an Endoscope Image. In: Taylor, C., Colchester, A. (eds.) MICCAI 1999. LNCS, vol. 1679, pp. 318–327. Springer, Heidelberg (1999)

Automatic Detection and Localization of da Vinci Tool Tips in 3D Ultrasound

Omid Mohareri, Mahdi Ramezani, Troy Adebar, Purang Abolmaesumi, and Septimiu Salcudean

Robotics and Control Laboratory, Department of Electrical and Computer Engineering, University of British Columbia, Vancouver, Canada

Abstract. Radical prostatectomy (RP) is viewed by many as the gold standard treatment for clinically localized prostate cancer. State of the art radical prostatectomy involves the da Vinci surgical system, a laparoscopic robot which provides the surgeon with excellent 3D visualization of the surgical site and improved dexterity over standard laparoscopic instruments. Given the limited field of view of the surgical site in Robot-Assisted Laparoscopic Radical Prostatectomy (RALRP), several groups have proposed the integration of Transrectal Ultrasound (TRUS) imaging in the surgical work flow to assist with the resection of prostate and sparing the Neuro-Vascular Bundle (NVB). Rapid and automatic registration of TRUS imaging coordinates to the da Vinci tools or camera is a critical component of this integration. We propose a fully automatic registration technique based on accurate and automatic localization of robot tool tips pressed against the air-tissue boundary of the prostate, in 3D TRUS. The detection approach uses a multi-scale filtering technique to uniquely identify and localize the tool tip in the ultrasound volume and could also be used to detect other surface fiducials in 3D ultrasound. Feasibility experiments using a phantom and two *ex vivo* tissue samples yield promising results with target registration error (defined as the root mean square distance of corresponding points after registration) of ($1.80~mm$) that proves the system's accuracy for registering 3D TRUS to the da Vinci surgical system.

Keywords: Robot-assisted surgery, da Vinci surgical robot, 3D ultrasound, fiducial detection.

1   Introduction

Laparoscopic surgery (also known as keyhole or minimally invasive surgery) has various advantages over traditional open surgery, including reduced blood loss, hospital stay, recovery time, and scar-tissue formation. Robot-assisted laparoscopic surgery using the da Vinci Surgical System (Intuitive Surgical, Sunnyvale, CA) is emerging as a new standard of treatment, particularly for urologic procedures such as radical prostatectomy. Augmented reality, implemented as the overlay of medical images data onto a stereoscopic camera view, is one research

P. Abolmaesumi et al. (Eds.): IPCAI 2012, LNAI 7330, pp. 22–32, 2012.
© Springer-Verlag Berlin Heidelberg 2012

concept aimed at offsetting the visual and haptic limitations of da Vinci laparoscopic surgery. The displayed data can come from several medical imaging modalities such as ultrasound [2,10], fluoroscopy, CT [10] and MRI, depending on the tissue types involved in the procedure [5,7]. All augmented reality systems must include algorithms for accurately registering medical images to camera images in real time.

A current augmented-reality-based research in this area involves registering intraoperative 3D ultrasound images of the prostate to the da Vinci stereoscopic camera view during robot-assisted laparoscopic radical prostatectomy (RALRP). A robotic system for Transrectal ultrasound (TRUS) imaging during RALRP is designed [1] and is being used to capture two-dimensional and three-dimensional B-mode and elastography data. A method for 3D ultrasound to stereoscopic camera registration through an air-tissue boundary [14] is used to register the TRUS images to the da Vinci camera. The same registration technique is also implemented to allow the TRUS robot to automatically track the da Vinci tool tips with the TRUS imaging planes to provide guidance without any distraction to the surgeon. A schematic of this approach and the prostate anatomy during RALRP is shown in Figure 1. This registration method uses da Vinci tool tips or other fiducials pressed against the air-tissue boundary and requires knowledge of the position of the tool tips/fiducials in the ultrasound frame in real time. The da Vinci API or the da Vinci camera are used to provide the location of the tool tips/fiducials in the da Vinci frame or the camera frame. Once fiducials are localized in both frames, the homogeneous transformation between them could be solved using a least squares method.

The process of localizing the da Vinci tool tips or the surface fiducials in 3D ultrasound volumes is done manually and involves scrolling through 2D slices of the volume, finding the 2D slice with the tool tip inside and selecting the approximate center of each fiducial through mouse positioning and clicking. While the overall registration technique is a success, the process of manual fiducial selection

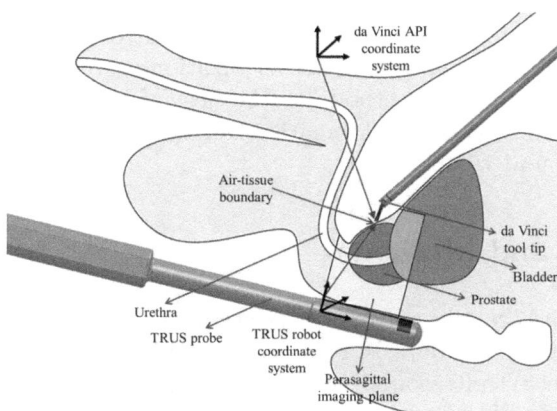

Fig. 1. Air-tissue boundary registration concept for automatic tool-tracking in RALRP

is time consuming and the interpretation of the fiducial centers in series of 2D
ultrasound images in the volume is subjective and varies from user to user. An
automatic fiducial localization algorithm would be easier to use than the manual
selection and also may help to avoid disrupting the surgical workflow, moving
the overall augmented reality and tool tracking systems further towards a real
time implementation. This work will address the problem of automatic da Vinci
tool tip localization in 3D TRUS but the detection algorithm could be easily
used for other types of surface fiducials.

Localization of surgical tools in 3D ultrasound has been addressed in a few
works [6,11], but to the best of authors' knowledge, there is no report on automatic tool tip localization in 3D Transrectal ultrasound. This problem can be
divided into two sub-problems: (i) automatically detecting the presence of the
tool tip in the ultrasound volume and finding its slice number, (ii) automatically locating the center of each detected tool tip in the 2D frame. Poon and
Rohling [12], in a study on calibration of 3D ultrasound probes (a separate and
unrelated type of calibration), used the centroid of an image region around a
user-supplied location to semi-automatically detect the center of each fiducial.
This simple concept solves the second sub-problem, but not the first. The goal of
this study is to recommend a method to target both of the above problems and
make the tool tip localization procedure fully automatic without compromising
the previously achieved registration accuracy $2.37 \pm 1.15\ mm$ [1].

A multi scale filtering technique based on second order Gaussian derivative
and a circular Hough transform is proposed and implemented for da Vinci too
tip localization in 3D ultrasound. A 3D mask is created based on the background
ultrasound volume (a volume that has been imaged before inserting the tool tip
into the tissue) and applied to the ultrasound volume that includes the tool
tip. This ultrasound volume is then filtered to find the edges representing the
candidate tip locations in the remaining part of the image. Eventually, the tip of
the tool is found by using a circular Hough transform. Hence, the tool location
is both determined in the ultrasound volume and inside its 2D frame. The same
method could be used to localize any surface fiducial pressed against the air-
tissue boundary. Experiments have been performed to evaluate the registration
accuracy using this automatic fiducial localization method and the results are
compared with the manual method. To the best of authors' knowledge, this is
the first implementation of an automatic algorithm for detecting da Vinci tools
inside 3D ultrasound volumes.

2   Material and Methods

Several key factors are relevant to the selection of a detection algorithm for this
problem. The ultrasound data is available in real time as a series of 2D images
generated by the 3D ultrasound transducer scanning the body. Although the
ultrasound considered in this study is three-dimensional, the actual volumes are
created by an off-line scan conversion algorithm and therefore, the detection algorithm must be applied to the sequence of 2D images creating the 3D volume.

The appearance of the target objects is fairly consistent. Ultrasound images of da Vinci tool tips pressed against air-tissue boundaries all contain similar features: strong horizontal lines from the air-tissue boundary and approximately circular areas of high-intensity from the tool tips themselves. The scale of the ultrasound volumes is fixed by the spatial resolution of the ultrasound transducer, so scale invariance is not required. Prostate surgeries will involve fairly consistent relative orientations of transducer and probe, so rotational invariance is likewise not required. Finally, the detection must be very rapid. In an ideal real time augmented reality system, the medical image data displayed in the surgeon's stereo view would be updated at a rate close to that of normal video (i.e. 30 frames per second) and therefore, a detection algorithm that can scan an entire volume in a few seconds is necessary to avoid disrupting the surgical work flow.

2.1 Automatic Detection Algorithm

In this study, the automatic extraction of da Vinci tool tips is done in four steps: masking, filtering, circle detecting and removing the false positives. A schematic of the first three steps of this method is shown in the diagram of Figure 3. The idea behind creating the mask is to detect the air tissue boundary and remove everything which lies below this line corresponding to the air part in the ultrasound image. Figure 2 shows an example image of da Vinci tool tip pressed against the air-tissue boundary of an *ex vivo* liver tissue. To create a 3D mask, first series of 2D images of the background volume have been filtered using a Hessian based Frangi vesselness filter [4]. In this filtering approach, the principal directions in which the maximum changes occur in the gradient vector of the underlying intensity in a small neighborhood are identified. Eigenvalue decomposition of the Hessian matrix can give these directions. Therefore, the Hessian matrix at each pixel of the image for a particular scale (σ) of the Gaussian derivative operator is computed. Then, the eigenvalue decomposition is used to extract two orthonormal directions. Based on the computed eigenvalues (λ_1, λ_2)

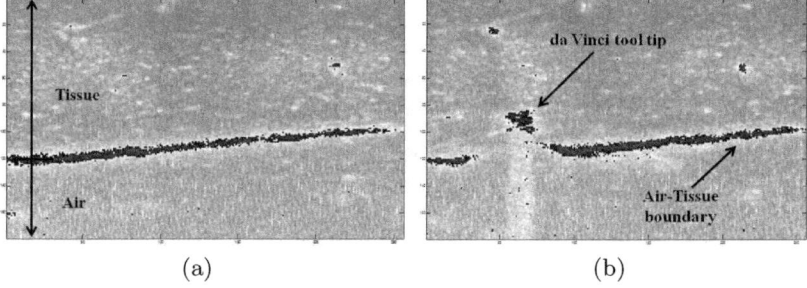

(a)   (b)

Fig. 2. (a) Example of an air-tissue boundary in an *ex vivo* liver phantom. (b) da Vinci tool tip pressed against an air-tissue boundary.

at each scale ($\Sigma = 1, 3, 5$) , a measure is defined as follows [4]:

$$S = \max_{\sigma \in \Sigma} S(\sigma) = \begin{cases} 0 & \text{if } \lambda_2 > 0 \\ \exp(\frac{R_b^2}{2\beta^2})(1 - \exp(-\frac{R_n^2}{2c^2})) & \text{if } \lambda_2 < 0 \end{cases} \tag{1}$$

$R_b = \frac{\lambda_1}{\lambda_2}$ is the blobness measure in 2D, and $R_n = \sqrt{\lambda_1^2 + \lambda_2^2}$ is a background or noise reduction term. R_b shows deviation from blob-like structures and R_n shows the presence of the structure using the fact that the magnitude of the derivatives (eigenvalues) is small in the background pixels. In this equation β is chosen as 0.5 and c is chosen to be the $\max_{x,y} R_n$. Images are further processed to remove the small areas of high intensity which are randomly scattered in the filtered image and are due to speckles. The image is first thresholded by a threshold obtained from the mean value of the intensities of pixels of the images. Next, parts that have less than M connected components are removed. M is a number obtained by trial and error for TRUS images. The remaining components, which represent the high intensity and relatively large areas corresponding to the tissue structures in the image, are dilated using morphological operators. To find the air-tissue boundary a line detection using Hough transform has been applied to the images. Lines with the minimum length of 30 and minimum gap of 15 pixels between them, have been extracted. A mask has been created using the

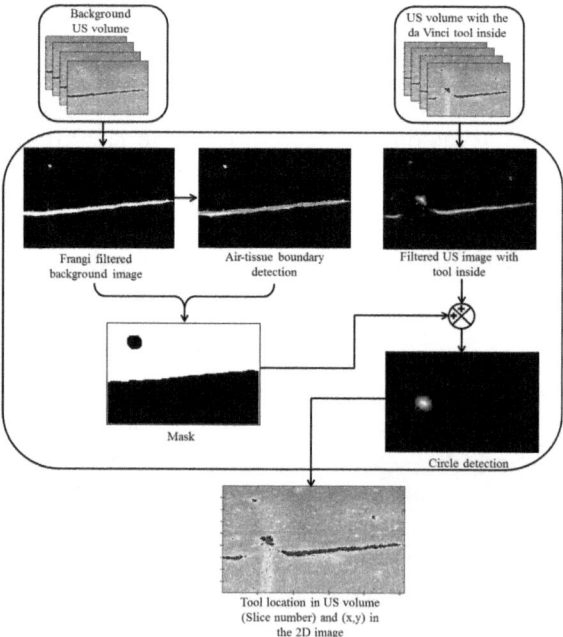

Fig. 3. The structure of the automatic tool detection algorithm. The background ultrasound volume and the volume with the tool inside are the inputs. Slice number and x,y position of the tool tip in the detected slice are the outputs.

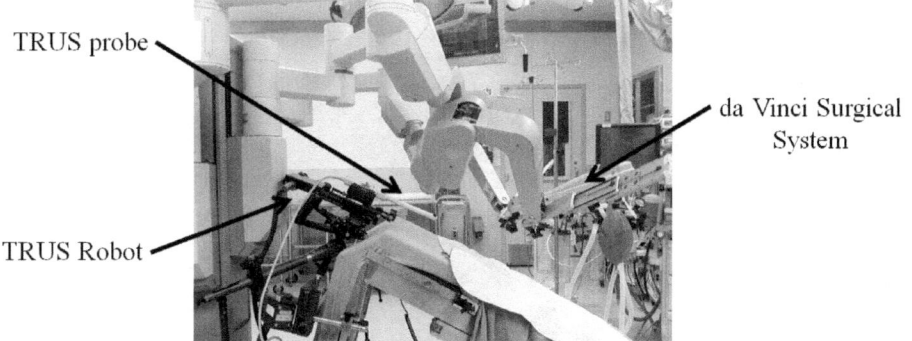

TRUS probe

da Vinci Surgical
System

TRUS Robot

Fig. 4. Experimental setup used for ultrasound imaging: TRUS robot and the da Vinci surgical system

detected air-tissue boundary and artifacts. The mask is responsible to remove regions corresponding to the artifacts and regions outside the tissue boundary.

After applying the mask to the 3D ultrasound volume, the Frangi filter is applied to the series of 2D images and the relatively large components are extracted. A circular Hough transform is applied to the obtained components to find circles with radius of approximately 5 pixels and minimum pixels of 20. The mean location of these circles in each 2D image is computed as candidates of the tool location. Next, a hierarchical clustering algorithm [9] is performed to find the group of candidates which are in adjacent slices, considering the fact that the tool tip can be seen in a couple of consecutive slices. Euclidean distance between the identified candidates has been used as a similarity measure and those which are close to each other are linked to create the cluster. The linkage function continues until an inconsistency coefficient reaches its threshold [8]. Using this approach false positively detected candidates will be removed due to the fact that false positives do not necessarily occur in adjacent slices. Once the cluster of 2D images that have the tool inside them are found, the middle slice in the cluster is chosen to be the output slice for the detection algorithm.

2.2 Experimental Setup for Ultrasound Image Acquisition

The robotic system shown in Figure 4, which is designed for intra-operative TRUS imaging during RALRP, is used for ultrasound image acquisition in this study. The system has three main parts: a robotic ultrasound probe manipulator (robot), an ultrasound machine with a biplane TRUS probe, and control and image processing software. Ultrasound images are captured using a parasagittal/transverse biplane TRUS probe in combination with a Sonix TABLET ultrasound machine (Ultrasonix Medical Corp., Richmond, Canada). 3D ultrasound volumes are collected by rotating the 2D imaging planes and automatically recording the encoder positions for each image. Software running on the ultrasound console is responsible for directing the robot movements and the ultrasound data acquisition. Currently, a

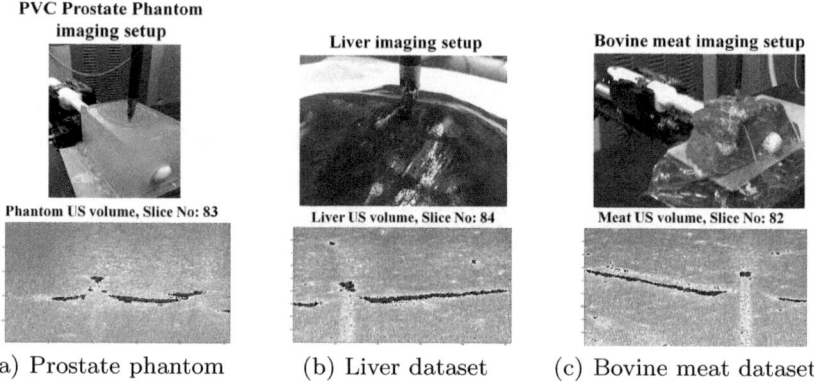

(a) Prostate phantom   (b) Liver dataset   (c) Bovine meat dataset

Fig. 5. Sample tool detection results for three different data sets

simple graphical user interface (GUI) is being used to allow the user to position the probe, and automatically collect 2D B-mode images and radio-frequency (RF) data while rotating from -40 to +40 degrees. A standard brachytherapy stabilizer arm (Micro-Touch 610-911; CIVCO Medical Solutions, Kalona, IA) is mounted to the operating table and the robot is installed on the stabilizer as it is shown in Figure 4.

3 Results

The proposed automatic tool detection method has been tested on three different acquired data sets: a custom-made PVC prostate phantom, an *ex vivo* liver and *ex vivo* bovine meat. Some sample results of the tool detection algorithm along with the testing configuration for each of the data sets are shown in Figure 5.

The rigid point registration technique proposed by Umeyama in [13], is used in this study to evaluate the automatic detection algorithm's performance. The manual fiducial localization process is replaced by the developed automatic localization algorithm, and the registration accuracy is re-calculated. Da Vinci tool tips are pressed against 12 different points on the air-tissue boundary of each of the three collected data-sets ($N_t = 12$) and its positions (x^0) in the ultrasound robot frame $\{O_0, C_0\}$ is calculated using our automatic detection algorithm. The da Vinci API is used to provide the location of the tool tips (x^1) in the da Vinci frame $\{O_1, C_1\}$.

For each registration experiment, N_f number of points ($N_f \geq 3$) are randomly picked from the total points collected for each tissue type and the rigid point registration method explained in [14] is used to compute the transformation between the frames T_0^1 to minimize the Fiducial Registration Error (FRE). FRE is computed as the root-mean-square of distances between corresponding fiducials after this registration. Next, the rest of the points in each data-set are assumed to be the target points and the calculated transformation is used to transform

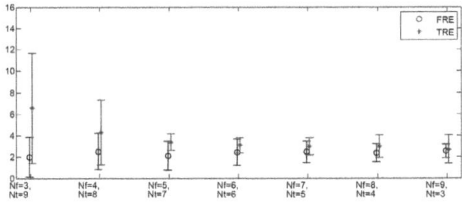

Fig. 6. FRE and TRE and their standard deviations for different numbers of fiducials (N_f) and target points(N_t)

them from the ultrasound robot frame to the da Vinci frame and the Target Registration Error (TRE) is estimated. Estimated TRE includes the real TRE and the target localization error (TLE). TRE is defined as the root-mean-square of distances between corresponding fiducials after registration, i.e., the distance between the localized position of each tool tip as transformed from the ultrasound robot space to da Vinci space and the position of that corresponding tool tip localized in the da Vinci space provided by the API. Because of the Fiducial Localization Error (FLE), the registration is inevitably inaccurate to some extent, and TRE is used as the available measure of registration error. Values of FRE and TRE are computed for different number of fiducials N_f chosen between the total points for each data-set N_t. The mean values of FRE and TRE and their standard deviations are then calculated for each combination of (N_f, N_t) for 100 iterations $(n = 100)$ and the results are plotted for the liver dataset in Figure 6. As it can be seen from Figure 6, as (N_f) increases, both mean and standard deviation of TRE decreases and based on this analysis, the number of fiducials suggested for this registration is $(N_f = 5)$. The mean and standard deviation values of the target registration error (TRE) for this number of fiducials and 100 iterations are reported in the anatomical frame of the patient in Table 1. Tool tip segmentation error is also calculated in (x, y, θ) directions. Three subjects were asked to independently identify the location of the tool in ultrasound images. The difference between the average user defined positions and the result of our algorithm, in addition to the inter-subject variations are calculated. For the liver dataset, automatic segmentation error is: $e(x, y) = 3.11 \pm 0.88\ mm$,

Table 1. Mean errors $(n = 100)$ between tool tip location and predicted location based on registration. Errors are presented in the anatomical frame of the patient, along the superior-inferior (e_{S-I}), medial-lateral (e_{M-L}) and anterior-posterior (e_{A-P}) axes.

	$TRE_{A-P}\ mm$	$TRE_{S-I}\ mm$	$TRE_{M-L}\ mm$	Mean TRE mm
Phantom	0.62 ± 0.31	1.29 ± 0.22	0.82 ± 0.24	1.80 ± 0.32
Liver	0.72 ± 0.83	2.65 ± 0.51	1.18 ± 0.54	3.33 ± 0.81
Bovine meat	1.90 ± 0.79	1.24 ± 0.34	3.51 ± 0.70	4.54 ± 0.88

$e(\theta) = 0.79° \pm 0.39°$ and the inter-subject variation is: $e(x, y) = 4.25 \pm 1.45 \ mm$, $e(\theta) = 2.05° \pm 0.8°$. For the pvc phantom dataset, automatic segmentation error is: $e(x, y) = 2.13 \pm 0.97 \ mm$, $e(\theta) = 0.67° \pm 0.34°$ and the inter-subject variation is: $e(x, y) = 3.65 \pm 0.88 \ mm$, $e(\theta) = 1.55° \pm 0.39°$. For the bovine meat dataset, automatic segmentation error is: $e(x, y) = 2.42 \pm 1.19 \ mm$, $e(\theta) = 0.68° \pm 0.48°$ and the inter-subject variation is: $e(x, y) = 3.13 \pm 0.88 \ mm$, $e(\theta) = 1.43° \pm 0.44°$.

4   Discussion

The overall average TRE previously reported using the manual fiducial localization of three fiducials on the PVC tissue phantom was $2.37 \pm 1.15 \ mm$. The overall average TRE using the automatic detection technique in this study is $1.80 \pm 0.32 \ mm$ for the recommended number of fiducial points, $N_f = 5$, on the PVC tissue phantom. As the number of fiducials is increased to 9, the TRE value reaches its minimum calculated value which is $1.61 \pm 0.39 \ mm$, which is consistent with the previously reported theoretical analysis [3]. To further evaluate the algorithm, experiments have been done on ex vivo liver and bovine meat which are more similar to the human prostate tissue. The minimum calculated TRE value is $2.86 \pm 1.40 \ mm$ for the liver and $4.15 \pm 0.61 \ mm$ for the bovine meat for picking 9 fiducials on the air-tissue boundary. According to these results, the automatic detection algorithm could yield the same registration accuracy as the manual detection method does, and it could also compensate for errors resulting from mis-interpretation of tool location in the ultrasound volume. The goal of tracking is to have the tool tips appear in the TRUS images and errors in the axial and lateral ultrasound directions are irrelevant as long as the tool tips are within the image boundaries. And because the thickness of the TRUS beam at the anterior surface of the prostate is on the order of millimeters, small errors in the elevational direction likely are not critical. We propose choosing five tool positions on the tissue surface, $N_f = 5$, both to achieve an acceptable registration error and to have a reasonable number of tissue poking repetitions during the surgical procedure. Because this registration technique is designed for RALRP procedure, it is recommended to choose two points on the prostate apex, one point on the mid-gland and two points on the prostate base. In this process, da Vinci tool is slightly pressed on the surface of the tissue at different locations. Hence, there won't be a significant movement in the organ and only the air-tissue boundary is moved about $2 - 3 \ mm$ at locations where the tool tip is placed. Also, only the tip of the tool (i.e., the area that touches the tissue) could be seen and detected in the ultrasound images. The instrument shaft could not be seen in the images and could not be used as an additional feature.

Replacing the process of manual detection of tool tips or surface fiducials in the ultrasound volume will accelerate the registration time and reduces the amount of surgical work-flow disruption. There will be no need for a sonographer to attend the surgery to find the tool tip in the ultrasound volume and the algorithm will reliably find the tool tips and send the points to the registration module to calculate the transformation. In addition, the results will not be dependent on the person who is choosing the points in the ultrasound volumes as it is the case in the manual detection.

5 Conclusions

In this study, we have addressed the problem of detecting da Vinci tool tips pressed against an air-tissue boundary, in a 3D ultrasound volume. A method based on multi-scale filtering and circle detection has been proposed. The tool tip localization accuracy is evaluated by analyzing the registration error between the TRUS robot frame and the da Vinci frame. Results show the equivalency of the proposed method and the previously reported manual detection procedure. As an overall comment on the proposed method, it is to be stressed that the method has a significant improving effect on both the duration,complexity and accuracy of the registration procedure. Future work will involve investigating *in vivo* studies to verify the accuracy and reliability of the proposed technique during RALRP procedure.

References

1. Adebar, T., Salcudean, S., Mahdavi, S., Moradi, M., Nguan, C., Goldenberg, L.: A Robotic System for Intra-operative Trans-Rectal Ultrasound and Ultrasound Elastography in Radical Prostatectomy. In: Taylor, R.H., Yang, G.-Z. (eds.) IPCAI 2011. LNCS, vol. 6689, pp. 79–89. Springer, Heidelberg (2011)
2. Cheung, C.L., Wedlake, C., Moore, J., et al.: Fusion of stereoscopic video and laparoscopic ultrasound for minimally invasive partial nephrectomy. In: Proceedings of SPIE Medical Imaging, vol. 7261, pp. 1–10 (2009)
3. Danilchenko, A., Fitzpatrick, J.M.: General approach to first-order error prediction in rigid point registration. IEEE Trans. on Medical Imaging 30(3), 679–693 (2011)
4. Frangi, A.F.: 3D model-based analysis of vascular and cardiac images (2001)
5. Fuchs, H., Livingston, M.A., Raskar, R., Keller, K., State, A., Crawford, J.R., Rademacher, P., Drake, S.H., Meyer, A.A.: Augmented Reality Visualization for Laparoscopic Surgery. In: Wells, W.M., Colchester, A.C.F., Delp, S.L. (eds.) MICCAI 1998. LNCS, vol. 1496, pp. 934–943. Springer, Heidelberg (1998)
6. Gaufillet, F., Liegbott, H., Uhercik, M., et al.: 3d ultrasound real-time monitoring of surgical tools. In: IEEE Ultrasonics Symposium (IUS), pp. 2360–2363 (2010)
7. Grimson, E., Leventon, M., Ettinger, G., Chabrerie, A., Ozlen, F., Nakajima, S., Atsumi, H., Kikinis, R., Black, P.: Clinical Experience with a High Precision Image-Guided Neurosurgery System. In: Wells, W.M., Colchester, A.C.F., Delp, S.L. (eds.) MICCAI 1998. LNCS, vol. 1496, pp. 63–73. Springer, Heidelberg (1998)
8. Guide, M.U.: The mathworks. Inc., Natick, MA 5 (1998)
9. Johnson, S.C.: Hierarchical clustering schemes. Psychometrika 32(3), 241–254 (1967)
10. Linte, C.A., Moore, J., Wiles, A.D., et al.: Virtual reality-enhanced ultrasound guidance: A novel technique for intracardiac interventions. Computer Aided Surgery 13(2), 82–94 (2008)
11. Novotny, P.M., Stoll, J.A., Vasilyev, N.V., Nido, P.J.D., Dupont, P.E., Zickler, T.E., Howe, R.D.: Gpu based real-time instrument tracking with three-dimensional ultrasound. Medical Image Analysis 11(5), 458–464 (2007)

12. Poon, T.C., Rohling, R.N.: Tracking a 3-d ultrasound probe with constantly visible fiducials. Ultrasound in Medicine & Biology 33(1), 152–157 (2007)
13. Umeyama, S.: Least-squares estimation of transformation parameters between two point patterns. IEEE Trans. on PAMI 13(4), 376–380 (1991)
14. Yip, M.C., Adebar, T.K., Rohling, R.N., Salcudean, S.E., Nguan, C.Y.: 3D Ultrasound to Stereoscopic Camera Registration through an Air-Tissue Boundary. In: Jiang, T., Navab, N., Pluim, J.P.W., Viergever, M.A. (eds.) MICCAI 2010. LNCS, vol. 6362, pp. 626–634. Springer, Heidelberg (2010)

Real-Time Methods for Long-Term Tissue Feature Tracking in Endoscopic Scenes

Michael C. Yip[1], David G. Lowe[2], Septimiu E. Salcudean[1],
Robert N. Rohling[1], and Christopher Y. Nguan[3]

[1] Electrical and Computer Engineering, University of British Columbia, Canada
[2] Computer Science Department, University of British Columbia, Canada
[3] Vancouver General Hospital, Vancouver, British Columbia, Canada

Abstract. Salient feature tracking for endoscopic images has been investigated in the past for 3D reconstruction of endoscopic scenes as well
as tracking of tissue through a video sequence. Recent work in the field
has shown success in acquiring dense salient feature profiling of the scene.
However, there has been relatively little work in performing long-term
feature tracking for capturing tissue deformation. In addition, real-time
solutions for tracking tissue features result in sparse densities, rely on re-
strictive scene and camera assumptions, or are limited in feature distinctiveness. In this paper, we develop a novel framework to enable long-term
tracking of image features. We implement two fast and robust feature algorithms, STAR and BRIEF, for application to endoscopic images. We
show that we are able to acquire dense sets of salient features at real-time
speeds, and are able to track their positions for long periods of time.

1 Introduction

There are many instances in which image guidance for minimally invasive surgery
requires tissue tracking in endoscopic video sequences in a robust manner. Tissue tracking provides an evaluation of tissue morphology and deformation *in-vivo*
over time, which can be important for tracking regions of interest such as vascu-
lature or lesions. When a medical image is registered to the stereoscopic cameras
for augmented reality, tissue tracking provides the knowledge of how the underlying tissues are moving such that the medical image can be moved accordingly.
This keeps anatomical features such as nerves and lesions in known locations
during surgical intervention, which can be critical in enabling the success of an
operation such as laparoscopic radical prostatectomy (LRP) [19]. In LRP, the
surgeon images an exposed prostate using transrectal ultrasound (TRUS) and
dissects it from the surrounding tissues prior to resection. Since contact is lost
between the prostate and the surrounding tissue after mobilization, it is important to maintain an image registration to the mobilized prostate in order to
perform resection within adequate surgical margins (1.9 ± 0.8 mm [19]).

While many tissue tracking methods have been employed that use fiducial
markers, most recent work uses image-based non-invasive techniques. Unlike natural scenes and urban environments, tissue images have poor color and textural

P. Abolmaesumi et al. (Eds.): IPCAI 2012, LNAI 7330, pp. 33–43, 2012.

distinctiveness, few edges and corners, are poorly illuminated, exhibit a great deal of specular reflection, and exhibit non-rigid deformation due to regular patient motion (e.g. heartbeat, breathing) as well as interactions with surgical instruments. Therefore, simple template-based tracking has been found to be limited in performance[12,15]. Others have used deformation functions [13] to capture real-time deformations of a beating heart, but require predictive models for heartbeat motion, frequent reinitializations to avoid drift, and are only able to capture low-order deformations. The most successful method for densely tracking tissue deformation so far is feature tracking. Work by [6,9,11,18,21] and references therein have shown that it is possible to find stable and uniquely identifiable features in tissue images. However, two areas of difficulty still exists:

Feature Management for Long-Term Tracking. A framework for managing features that enter and exit an endoscopic scene is necessary to maintain long-term stable tracking. Despite the successes of Simultaneous Localization and Mapping methods for long-term tracking, they are suitable for natural scenes and urban environments and predominantly rely on camera pose estimation, assuming that scene features generally only move due to camera motion [20,21]. Due to patient movement (breathing, heartbeat) and surgical instrument interactions with tissues, these methods are limited in their application here. Therefore, a long-term feature tracking method, one that minimizes drift without estimating camera pose, and can track features temporarily lost between frames, is an important contribution.

Speed. Features with high saliency, such as the Scale Invariant Feature Transform (SIFT) [5], have been effective at producing dense, stable features [6,10,20,21], but are unable to run at real-time speeds. Computationally fast features (e.g. Shi-Tomasi [16], FAST [14]) have only been able to generate sparse sets of trackable points in real-time operation[8]. GPU implementations have been limited and have yet to achieve real-time speeds at high-definition, and still rely on some CPU computation where GPU-acceleration is deemed not effective [17]. Therefore, an interesting research question is: are we able to perform high-density feature tracking at real-time speeds?

In this paper, we will describe a novel long-term tissue tracking strategy that is capable of capturing a dense map of tissue deformations within endoscopic images. Using two relatively new salient feature algorithms (CenSuRE[1] and BRIEF[2]), we are able to achieve real-time (greater than 10Hz) speeds while maintaining high resolution tracking of tissue deformation for extended periods of time. Furthermore, we show that this can be applied to stereoscopic scenes for describing and tracking 3D tissue surface profiles.

2   Methods

2.1   Salient Features

We propose the use of two relatively new feature detectors: a modified version of the Center Surrounded Extremas (CenSuRE) feature detector [1] called STAR [22], and the Binary Robust Independent Elementary Features (BRIEF) [2].

Mikolojaczyk and Schmid [7] found that the most salient image features found in computer vision literature were derived from the Laplacian of Gaussian (LoG). Where SIFT uses a Difference of Gaussians to estimate the LoG, CenSuRE uses a bi-level center-surrounded square kernel, where pixel values within the kernel are multiplied by either +1 or -1 (Figure 1a). These kernels are applied over pyramidal scale space at all locations to find local extrema that represent salient features. The extrema are then filtered using a scale-adapted Harris measure to eliminate weak responses, and line suppression is performed by evaluating a second moment matrix, and discarding those features that have a large ratio between principle curvatures. The STAR feature detector [22] that we will be using is a modification of the CenSuRE detector by using a star shaped kernel (an overlay of a 0 deg and a 45 deg oriented CenSuRE kernel), in order to better estimate the LoG (Figure 1b). Given that these center-surround kernels are simply addition and subtraction summations, they can be computed extremely efficiently using integral images. The output of the STAR detector will be the salient locations and scales of patches in the image.

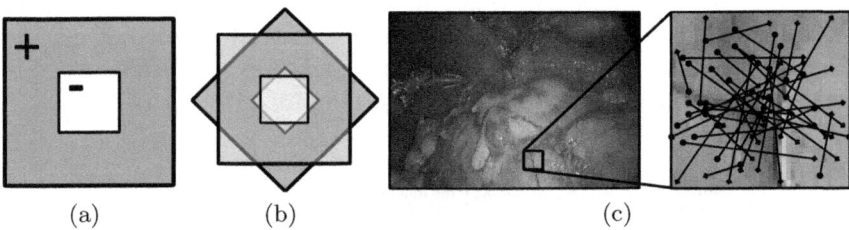

(a)   (b)   (c)

Fig. 1. (a) bi-level center-surround kernel constructed using integral images, and, (b) the STAR kernel, and (c) example of a BRIEF kernel

In order to track features from one frame to the next, we use the BRIEF [2] descriptor to describe a characteristically-scaled patch centered about each STAR location. For each STAR location, N pairs of points in an $S \times S$ square region are chosen at random, with the condition that the probability of choosing a point is equal to an isotropic Gaussian distribution centered about the STAR location (Figure 1c). A descriptor vector of length N is built to describe the patch, where the ith element is either 0 (if, for the ith pair, the pixel intensity of the first point is higher than that of the second point) or 1 (otherwise). This creates a binary vector that can be used to uniquely identify each feature. Feature matching is performed by calculating the Hamming distance between two feature descriptors. Following the formulation provided in [2], we use a patch size of $S = 25$ and vector length of $N = 256$.

There are a number of reasons as to why we chose to combine both STAR and BRIEF (STAR+BRIEF) to describe a single salient feature. Both methods evaluate patch-locations for saliency, and by extracting BRIEF features at characteristic scales of the STAR locations, STAR+BRIEF features can be made scale-invariant. STAR's approximation of the LoG can be well described by the isotropic Gaussian-distributed pixel comparison vector of a BRIEF feature. Finally, both methods are fast to compute. Performance comparisons of STAR and BRIEF to popular feature detectors can be found in their original papers [1,2].

2.2   Long-Term Feature Tracking

A salient feature tracking framework for long-term tracking is developed. As opposed to other suggested frameworks for feature tracking for endoscopic video [21,20], our method does not use camera pose estimation and feature location reprojection to estimate scene movement. Rather, we allow each feature to move independently and use spatial and temporal filters to remove tracking errors, and we allow features to be lost temporarily and found in subsequent frames.

Temporal Tissue Tracking. A visual flowchart of the proposed tissue tracking framework is presented in Figure 2. We begin by capturing an image from the surgical camera, and performing a pre-processing filter with a 3 × 3 Gaussian smoothing kernel. We then extract the image features from the current frame (Figure 2B) and match them to features found in previous frames (Figure 2C). A list of features is maintained, where previous features that are matched have their locations and descriptors updated, and features that were not matched in the current frame are added to the list. Finally, features that are matched below a certain percentage of frames are discarded (empirically set to 40%).

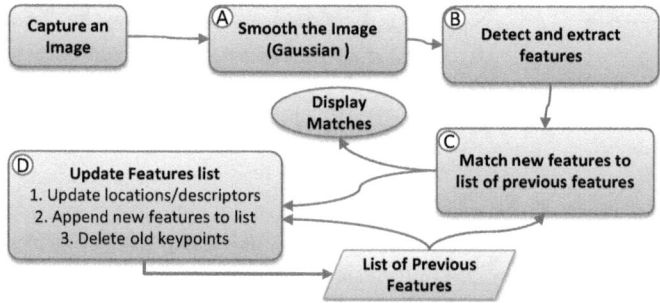

Fig. 2. Flowchart of the proposed feature tracking framework on a single image

There are a number of filters that are applied to improve feature matching accuracy. A feature is defined as $f(x, y, k)$, where x and y represent its pixel location in the original image, and k represents its characteristic scale. Given two feature lists (1 and 2), the ith feature from list 1, f_i, and the jth feature from list 2, f_j, we only perform descriptor comparisons on a subset of features.

- *Physical Proximity:* Since we do not expect large feature movement between consecutive frames, our search space is limited by

$$|x_i - x_j| < \delta_x \text{ and } |y_i - y_j| < \delta_y. \tag{1}$$

where δ_x and δ_y is the range of the search space.

- *Scale Similarity:* We do not expect significant changes in feature sizes between consecutive frames, and therefore limit our search space to

$$|log(k_i/k_j)| < \kappa, \qquad (2)$$

where κ is the maximum allowable ratio of feature scales.

- *Descriptor Distance Ratio:* We measure the confidence of feature matches by comparing the descriptor distance of the best match, d_{first}, to the descriptor distance of the second best match, d_{second}, and only take matches if

$$d_{first}/d_{second} < \lambda, \qquad (3)$$

where λ is the maximum allowable ratio between the descriptor distances.

A set of matched features will provide a dense mapping of tissue movement within the scene. Matches that move in significantly different directions than the local tissue movement can be rejected. This is performed by checking the movement of each matched feature against its nearest neighbors (matched features within a Euclidean distance of 20% of the image width).

Given a set of two neighboring feature locations in frame n, $Q_{1,n} = \{x_{1,n}, y_{1,n}\}$ and $Q_{2,n} = \{x_{2,n}, y_{2,n}\}$, and their matched locations in the previous frame, $Q_{1,n-1} = \{x_{1,n-1}, y_{1,n-1}\}$ and $Q_{2,n-1} = \{x_{2,n-1}, y_{2,n-1}\}$, we consider their movements to be significantly different if

$$\left| log\left(\frac{\delta x_1^2 + \delta y_1^2}{\delta x_2^2 + \delta y_2^2} \right) \right| > \gamma, \qquad (4)$$

where $\{\delta x_1, \delta y_1\} = \{x_{1,n} - x_{1,n-1}, y_{1,n} - y_{1,n-1}\}$ and $\{\delta x_2, \delta y_2\} = \{x_{2,n} - x_{2,n-1}, y_{2,n} - y_{2,n-1}\}$, and where γ represents the maximum allowable ratio of squared distances of movements between the neighboring features. Furthermore, the directions of their movements are considered to be significantly different if

$$\Delta\theta = acos\left(\frac{\delta x_1 \cdot \delta x_2 + \delta y_1 \cdot \delta y_2}{\sqrt{\delta x_1^2 + \delta y_1^2}\sqrt{\delta x_2^2 + \delta y_2^2}} \right) > \epsilon, \qquad (5)$$

where ϵ is the maximum allowable difference in the direction of movement.

Matched features that move within ϵ and γ for more than 70% of neighboring features are accepted. We check ϵ and γ only if there is a temporal displacement of 5 pixels for each match, since the resolution of ϵ and γ decreases significantly within a Euclidean distance of 5 pixels, making these filters less effective.

Stereoscopic Tracking. Our proposed tracking algorithm can be extended to track features in 3D coordinate space. Features from a left and right channel of a stereo-endoscope are matched in order to triangulate the features' locations in 3D. The matching between features in stereoscopic channels can be filtered using the same methods as above (Equations 1, 2 and 3). Since stereo-triangulation does not take into account temporal movement, neighborhood feature movement (Equations 4 and 5) are unnecessary for stereoscopic matching.

We use one channel for temporal tracking, and the tracked features are then matched against features found in the other channel for 3D localization; we note that in the future, tracking both channels can be used for outlier rejection.

3   Experimental Setup

Table 1 describes the parameters of our tissue tracking framework. $\kappa = \log(2.0)$ is chosen to search within an octave scale of a feature, and $\kappa = \log(\sqrt{2.0})$ reflects smaller changes in scale between stereo channels; δ's are chosen assuming that features move relatively small distances between frames and between stereoscopic channels. $\lambda = 0.5$ chooses feature matches that have under half the descriptor distance of the next best match. $\gamma = 2\log(1.5)$ and $\epsilon = \pi/18$ were chosen to restrict features bundles to smooth, consistent motion, characteristic of tissue.

Four measures were used to evaluate the efficacy of STAR+BRIEF and the long-term feature tracking strategy: (a) the number of features found per frame, (b) the percentage of these features that are matched to ones in previous frames, (c) the persistence of features in subsequent frames (d) and the algorithm speed.

We investigated the tracking algorithm's ability on four endoscopic videos involving different *in-vivo* tissue movement:

Translation: Abdominal cavity after inflation. Surgeon moves the endoscopic camera to approximate translation. (1050 frames, 480×640 pixels).

Rotation: Abdominal cavity after inflation. Surgeon moves the endoscopic camera to approximate rotation. (710 frames, 480×640 pixels).

Series: Abdominal cavity after inflation. Surgeon moves the endoscopic camera to approximate a series of movements involving translation and scaling with slight rotations. (1200 frames, 480×650 pixels)

Heartbeat: Open-chest procedure with an exposed heart. Significant surgical clamps footprint in the image. A stationary camera images a heartbeat. (650 frames, 720×576 pixels).

These videos, acquired by Imperial College London, are available at `http://ham lyn.doc.ic.ac.uk/vision/`

Table 1. Parameters for temporal and stereoscopic matching

Parameter	Symbol	Value (Temporal)	Value(Stereo)
Scale Threshold	κ	$\log(2.0)$	$\log(\sqrt{(2)})$
Local Area Threshold	δ	$0.2*$image_width	$0.5*$image_width on x-axis $0.05*$image_height in y-axis
Descriptor Distance Ratio	λ	0.5	0.5
Difference in movements	γ	$2 * \log(1.5)$	N/A
Difference in angles	ϵ	$\pi/18$	N/A

4   Results

Figure 3a,b shows two example (Series and Heartbeat videos) of STAR+BRIEF features that are tracked temporally over time. The number of features extracted by the STAR+BRIEF framework fully describe the deformation of the scene. The average number of features tracked are shown in Figure 3c. Figure 3d shows that the STAR+BRIEF framework is able to match 90% of its features from frame to frame for general cases, and over 50% can be matched stereoscopically for 3D localization. Matches were visually inspected and nearly all matches were found to correctly track a correct physical location. We found that fewer features were tracked in the heartbeat video; we believe this can be attributed to the greater degree of specular reflection and significant occlusion from blood, and also the systolic action of the heart, which exhibits frequencies higher than 100Hz that cannot be adequately captured in the endoscopic cameras with conventional framerates. Furthermore, slight discrepancies in triggering during steroscopic frame-grabbing can account for significant movement between stereo channels.

Figure 3e shows a histogram of the percentage of subsequent frames in which features are matched. The histograms are cumulative, where the first column (40% to 50% persistence) is the total number of features being continuously tracked by long-term tracking framework. Features below 40% persistence were not stable and therefore were discarded. The number of features continuously tracked over increasing percentage of frames is fairly linear for general motion. Heartbeat motion shows less features being tracked continuously, and a non-linear dropoff in persistence of features due to the lower stability of the features from dynamic motion, specular reflection and blood occlusion.

Figure 3f shows the speed of our tracking framework with the STAR+BRIEF method. We show that the our long-term tracking framework is able to process sequences above 10Hz and is capable of performing stereoscopic matching and 3D deformation tracking at a fraction of the total tracking time. The heartbeat video, due to the higher resolution and increased specular reflection and occlusion, identified many more features than other videos that were unstable and therefore required significantly higher computation effort than other videos.

Figure 4 shows a sample of the tracking of a feature in the Series video, which involves translation, scaling, and some rotation. A useful method for getting a sense of the aversion to drift, given that we do not have a ground-truth source, is forward-backward tracking [3] shown in Figure 4a, where we track a feature both forwards and backwards in time. Since our long-term feature tracking framework is history-dependent and therefore behaves differently moving in forwards and backwards time, it can be seen that the feature location does not drift. Figure 4b shows the feature location at different timesteps, indicating its stability throughout the sequence of motions.

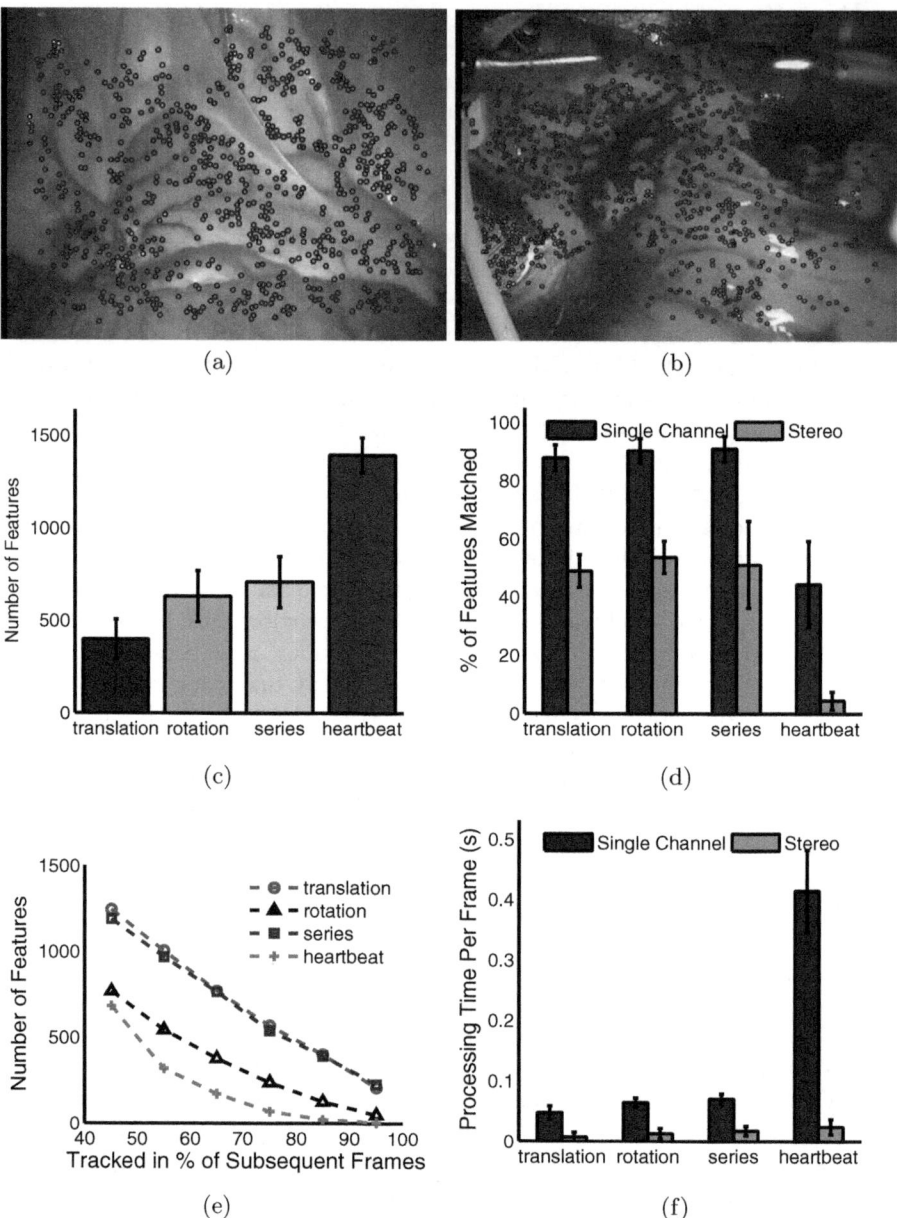

(a)   (b)

(c)   (d)

(e)   (f)

Fig. 3. (a,b) Sample feature set identified in the Series and Heartbeat sequences respectively. (c) Number of Features found per frame; (d) % of features in the current frame that are matched to previous features (blue) and % of features matched stereoscopically (orange); (e)The number of features that are found in % of subsequent frames. The graph is cumulative such that the number of features drops off as the % of matching in subsequent frames increases. (f) Time required for a complete cycle of the feature tracking framework (blue) and the amount of time required for stereoscopic matching (orange).

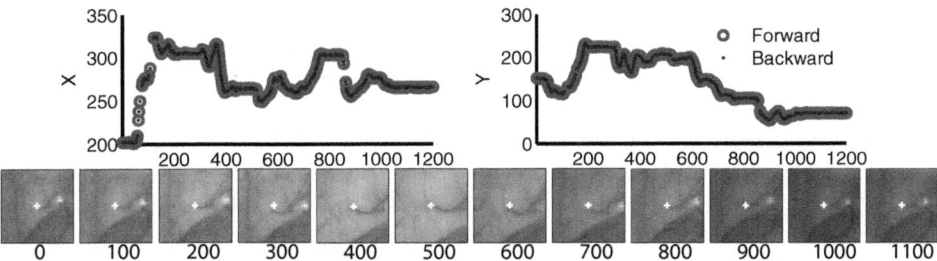

Fig. 4. A STAR+BRIEF feature being tracked over time (1200 frames). Top: tracking performed in both a forward and a backward time direction. Graph shows X and Y coordinates as a function of time. Bottom: a 50 × 50 pixel window centered about the feature location at every 100 frames.

5   Discussion

We have presented a novel framework for long-term tracking of endoscopic tissue scenes. This framework uses salient features for populating the endoscopic images in order to track the deformation of tissue at high densities. We have shown that by using two new, efficient feature algorithms, CenSuRE/STAR and BRIEF, we are able to achieve both high density tracking on standard definition video for long-periods of time at real-time (greater than 10 Hz) speeds. Other fast feature detectors, as well as GPU-accelerated feature tracking could also be used to achieve fast and dense feature tracking under this framework.

The performance of the algorithm is not reliant on a rigid scene or camera pose estimation and therefore can handle scene deformations, as tissue features are being tracked individually and therefore can describe complex deformations. However, in the case of significant high-frequency deformations (e.g. beating heart), the feature-based approach must widen its search space between frames in expectation of large dynamic movements of individual features. A reduction of the effects of specular reflection and blood occlusion are required to improve tracking, and several strategies can be used such as intensity thresholding and interpolation [4]. In the case of the beating heart, other strategies besides feature tracking, such as the ones presented in [13] can be more effective. Further efforts to handle specular reflection effects and to track instrument occlusion will help enable the long-term tracking strategy to track tissue through an entire surgery.

Given the long-term tissue feature tracking strategy we defined, it may be possible to maintain a registered medical image to endoscopic cameras by tracking the underlying tissue movements; this will provide the surgeon the ability to localize sub-surface tissue features such as nerves and lesions for better surgical guidance. Furthermore, the ability to acquire 3D tracking of dense feature maps may enable a surface-to-feature based registration method, such that the ability to register and maintain a medical image to tissues in the endoscopic cameras can be effectively streamlined. Future work will be to investigate the efficacy of registering and maintaining a medical image to the tissues seen in the laparoscopic cameras, with the motivation of improving surgical guidance in LRP, where the dissection of the prostate from the surrounding neurovascular bundle must be performed within narrow margins (1.9 ± 0.8 mm [19]).

Acknowledgments. The authors wish to thank NSERC and the CIHR Knowledge Translation Fund for supporting this work, as well as Professor Guang-Zhong Yang and the Hamlyn Centre for Robotic Surgery at Imperial College of London for open access to their *in-vivo* data sets. Research support from the C.A. Laszlo Chair held by Professor Salcudean is gratefully acknowledged.

References

1. Agrawal, M., Konolige, K., Blas, M.: CenSurE: Center Surround Extremas for Realtime Feature Detection and Matching. In: Forsyth, D., Torr, P., Zisserman, A. (eds.) ECCV 2008, Part IV. LNCS, vol. 5305, pp. 102–115. Springer, Heidelberg (2008)
2. Calonder, M., Lepetit, V., Strecha, C., Fua, P.: BRIEF: Binary Robust Independent Elementary Features. In: Daniilidis, K., Maragos, P., Paragios, N. (eds.) ECCV 2010. LNCS, vol. 6314, pp. 778–792. Springer, Heidelberg (2010)
3. Kalal, Z., Mikolajczyk, K., Matas, J.: Forward-backward error: Automatic detection of tracking failures. In: IEEE Int. C. Pattern Recognition, pp. 2756–2759 (2010)
4. Lo, B., Chung, A., Stoyanov, D., Mylonas, G., Yang, G.-Z.: Real-time intra-operative 3d tissue deformation recovery. In: I. S. Biomedical Imaging, pp. 1387–1390 (2008)
5. Lowe, D.G.: Distinctive image features from scale-invariant keypoints. Int. J. Computer Vision 60, 91–110 (2004)
6. Luó, X., Feuerstein, M., Reichl, T., Kitasaka, T., Mori, K.: An Application Driven Comparison of Several Feature Extraction Algorithms in Bronchoscope Tracking During Navigated Bronchoscopy. In: Liao, H., Edwards, P.J., Pan, X., Fan, Y., Yang, G.-Z. (eds.) MIAR 2010. LNCS, vol. 6326, pp. 475–484. Springer, Heidelberg (2010)
7. Mikolajczyk, K., Schmid, C.: A performance evaluation of local descriptors. IEEE T. Pattern Anal. 27, 1615–1630 (2005)
8. Mountney, P., Stoyanov, D., Davison, A., Yang, G.-Z.: Simultaneous Stereoscope Localization and Soft-Tissue Mapping for Minimal Invasive Surgery. In: Larsen, R., Nielsen, M., Sporring, J. (eds.) MICCAI 2006. LNCS, vol. 4190, pp. 347–354. Springer, Heidelberg (2006)
9. Mountney, P., Lo, B., Thiemjarus, S., Stoyanov, D., Zhong-Yang, G.: A Probabilistic Framework for Tracking Deformable Soft Tissue in Minimally Invasive Surgery. In: Ayache, N., Ourselin, S., Maeder, A. (eds.) MICCAI 2007, Part II. LNCS, vol. 4792, pp. 34–41. Springer, Heidelberg (2007)
10. Mountney, P., Yang, G.-Z.: Soft Tissue Tracking for Minimally Invasive Surgery: Learning Local Deformation Online. In: Metaxas, D., Axel, L., Fichtinger, G., Székely, G. (eds.) MICCAI 2008, Part II. LNCS, vol. 5242, pp. 364–372. Springer, Heidelberg (2008)
11. Mountney, P., Stoyanov, D., Yang, G.-Z.: Three-dimensional tissue deformation recovery and tracking. IEEE Signal Processing Magazine 27, 14–24 (2010)

12. Ortmaier, T., Groeger, M., Boehm, D., Falk, V., Hirzinger, G.: Motion estimation in beating heart surgery. IEEE T. Biomed. Eng. 52(10), 1729–1740 (2005)
13. Richa, R., Bo, A. P., Poignet, P.: Towards robust 3D visual tracking for motion compensation in beating heart surgery. Med. Image Anal. 15(3), 302-315 (2011)
14. Rosten, E., Drummond, T.: Machine Learning for High-Speed Corner Detection. In: Leonardis, A., Bischof, H., Pinz, A. (eds.) ECCV 2006. LNCS, vol. 3951, pp. 430–443. Springer, Heidelberg (2006)
15. Sauvee, M., Noce, A., Poignet, P., Triboulet, J., Dombre, E.: Three-dimensional heart motion estimation using endoscopic monocular vision system: From artificial landmarks to texture analysis. Biomed. Signal Process. Control 2(3), 199–207 (2007)
16. Shi, J., Tomasi, C.: Good features to track. In: IEEE Int. C. Computer Vision and Pattern Recognition, pp. 593–600 (1994)
17. Sinha, S. N., Frahm, J.-M., Pollefeys, M., Genc, Y.: Gpu-based video feature tracking and matching. In: Workshop on Edge Computing Using New Commodity Architectures, Technical Report (2006)
18. Stoyanov, D., Mylonas, G.P., Deligianni, F., Darzi, A., Yang, G.-Z.: Soft-Tissue Motion Tracking and Structure Estimation for Robotic Assisted MIS Procedures. In: Duncan, J.S., Gerig, G. (eds.) MICCAI 2005. LNCS, vol. 3750, pp. 139–146. Springer, Heidelberg (2005)
19. Ukimura, O., Gill, I., Desai, M.O.: Real-time transrectal ultrasonography during laparoscopic radical prostatectomy. Journal of Urology 172(1), 112–118 (2004)
20. Wang, H., Mirota, D., Ishii, M., Hager, G.: Robust motion estimation and structure recovery from endoscopic image sequences with an adaptive scale kernel consensus estimator. In: Int. C. Computer Vision and Pattern Recognition, pp. 1–7 (2008)
21. Wengert, C., Cattin, P.C., Duff, J.M., Baur, C., Székely, G.: Markerless Endoscopic Registration and Referencing. In: Larsen, R., Nielsen, M., Sporring, J. (eds.) MICCAI 2006. LNCS, vol. 4190, pp. 816–823. Springer, Heidelberg (2006)
22. Willow Garage. Star detector, http://pr.willowgarage.com/wiki/star_detector

A Closed-Form Differential Formulation for Ultrasound Spatial Calibration

Mohammad Najafi, Narges Afsham, Purang Abolmaesumi, and Robert Rohling

University of British Columbia, Vancouver, BC, Canada
rohling@ece.ubc.ca

Abstract. *Purpose*: Calibration is essential in tracked freehand 3D ultrasound (US) to find the spatial transformation from the image coordinates to the reference coordinate system. Calibration accuracy is especially important in image-guided interventions. *Method*: We introduce a new mathematical framework that substantially improves the US calibration accuracy. It achieves this by using accurate measurements of axial differences in 1D US signals of a multi-wedge phantom, in a closed-form solution. *Results*: We report a point reconstruction accuracy of 0.3 *mm* using 300 independent measurements. *Conclusion*: The measured calibration errors significantly outperform the currently reported calibration accuracies.

1   Introduction

Navigation based on preoperative images usually incorporates significant registration error, especially as surgery or therapy progresses. Over the past decade, intra-operative ultrasound navigation has become a rapidly emerging technique in many procedures including neurosurgery, orthopaedic surgery and radiation therapy. Being non-invasive, relatively inexpensive, and real-time makes ultrasound (US) a valuable tool in image-guided surgeries and therapies. By attaching a position sensor to a conventional 2D US probe, 3D images can be constructed. The main challenge of this *"freehand imaging"* is to precisely locate US image pixels with respect to sensors on the transducer which is referred to as the calibration process. In this process, the objective is to determine the spatial transform between US image coordinates and the fixed coordinate system, define by the tracker on the transducer housing.

Improper or poor probe calibration has been reported as one of the major contributors to the final accuracy of ultrasound neuronavigation [1]. For example, during US-guided resection of a liver tumor, the surgeon relies on ultrasound volumes for accurate orientation with respect to the tumor. To provide more safety with respect to tumor-free resection margins and preserve vessels close to the tumor, the ultrasound system has to be calibrated accurately [2].

Over the last two decades, many approaches for calibration of 2D and 3D US have been investigated [3,4]. Examples are single wall [5], hand-eye coordination [6] and the double N-wire [7]. The most accurate calibration techniques image an artificial object, known as a phantom, with known geometrical parameters,

P. Abolmaesumi et al. (Eds.): IPCAI 2012, LNAI 7330, pp. 44–53, 2012.

combining the prior knowledge of the phantom with its US images to solve for the calibration parameters. Despite numerous efforts, the best reported accuracies are in the order of 1 to 2 *mm*.

The limiting factor is the accurate, absolute localization of phantom features in B-mode images, which appear blurred due to the finite resolution and noise of US. Furthermore, many existing calibration methods use iterative optimization techniques to determine the calibration parameters, which are subject to sub-optimal local minima. Other factors, such as tracking accuracy and image formation errors due to speed of sound variation, refraction and finite beam width also contribute to the accuracy of calibration methods based on absolute measurements. It is worth noting that closed-form calibration from two different poses using hand-eye coordination has been proposed for measurements of relative shifts of features between images [6]. Relative measurements may have an inherent advantage, but the challenge in that method is to accurately estimate the relative 3D poses of the 2D ultrasound images.

In this paper, we propose a novel ultrasound calibration technique that alleviates many of these issues and provides substantially higher calibration accuracy. The new technique is closest to previous calibration research using wedge phantoms [6,8]. In particular, the technique uses differential measurements within the same image rather than absolute ones of phantom features in the image. Advancements in recent years on differential measurements for ultrasound motion tracking enable accurate measurements of relative phantom feature locations. This accuracy could be as high as a few microns when RF ultrasound is used [9]. The differential measurements mostly eliminate the need for absolute localization of the calibration phantom features, which has been a prominent factor in limiting the accuracy of current calibration techniques. The proposed technique also solves for variations in speed of sound and image skew. The solution to the calibration parameters also has a closed-form, which eliminates the need for an iterative optimization method.

2   Materials and Methods

The proposed calibration method is based on scanning a multi-wedge phantom that can be simply described as five different planes (Fig. 1b). The purpose of the planes is that echoes from different portions of a plane will have similar RF signatures, which enhances the ability to perform differential measurements within an image. We utilized the Field II simulation package to determine suitable angles of the planes based on image quality. In order to track the coordinate system of the phantom, four optical active markers are attached to the phantom. Also, two non-overlapping N-wires with known geometry and location relative to the planes are incorporated in the same phantom. The N-wire assembly provides an independent setup to evaluate the calibration accuracy Fig. 1a. The phantom was precisely manufactured with the Objet30 desktop 3D printer (Objet Inc., Billerica, MA, USA) to 28 μm precision and relatively low cost (< \$200).

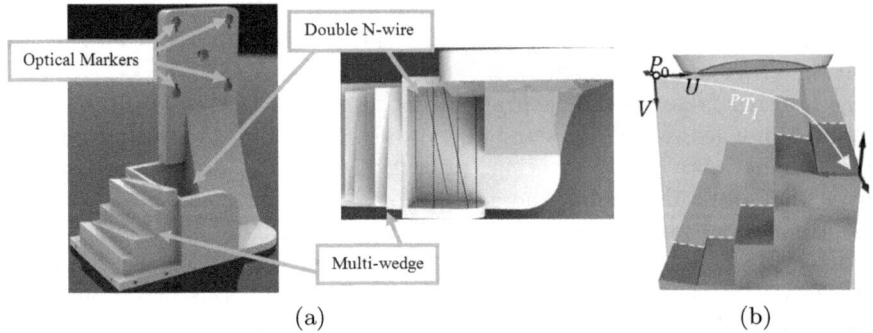

Fig. 1. (a) Multi-wedge phantom with four optical markers for tracking and an attached double N-wire phantom (b) The multi-wedge phantom comprising of five different planes. The dashed line shows the ultrasound image intersection line segments.

The calibration experimental setup consists of a SonixTOUCH ultrasound machine (Ultrasonix Medical Corporation, Richmond, BC, Canada), a L14 − 5, 10 MHz linear 2D ultrasound transducer, and an Optotrak Certus optical tracker (Northern Digital Inc, Waterloo, Ontario, Canada).

In our experiments, the coordinate systems of the phantom and the ultrasound transducer are measured by tracking the optical markers mounted on them (Fig. 2a). Therefore transformation from the phantom to the transducer coordinate can be found ($^T T_P$). The calibration goal is to find transformation from the image to the transducer coordinate ($^T T_I$). To solve that, we must calculate the image to phantom transformation ($^P T_I$).

Each plane appears as a line in the ultrasound image (dashed lines in Fig. 1b). The slope and intercept of these lines depend on the pose of the ultrasound image relative to the phantom. In fact, the goal is to find the pose of the US image ($^P T_I$) by measuring these line features in the ultrasound image. For this reason, a closed-form algorithm has been developed to estimate the calibration parameters using a single ultrasound image given the geometrical model of the phantom.

2.1   Mathematical Framework and Notations

We define the calibration phantom with the equations of five different planes. Here, we assume that the normal vector (n_i) and a point (Q_i) of each plane is known in a common coordinate system (i.e. the phantom coordinates).

The unknown transformation from the image to the phantom frame, ($^P T_I$), can be defined from two free vectors U and V and a point P_0 as follows (Fig. 2b). U is a unit vector in the direction passing through the center of array elements (lateral) and V is a unit vector in the direction of ultrasound beam (axial). These two vectors are usually assumed to be perpendicular but here we do not impose this assumption for a more general solution. P_0 is the origin of imaging plane in the phantom coordinates and is the translation vector in $^P T_I$.

2.2 Rotation Parameters

We first estimate the rotation parameters in $^P T_I$ by calculating vectors $\boldsymbol{U}$, $\boldsymbol{V}$ and S_y and then, by solving for P_0 we determine the translation parameters. Each pixel (x_1, y_1) of the image can be described in the phantom coordinates as:

$$P = P_0 + S_x x_1 \boldsymbol{U} + S_y y_1 \boldsymbol{V}. \tag{1}$$

Considering the pixels on the line appeared in the ultrasound image from the intersection of the phantom's i^{th} plane and the ultrasound image plane, they should satisfy the plane equation for plane i (Fig. 2b):

$$[P_0 + S_x x_1 \boldsymbol{U} + S_y y_1 \boldsymbol{V} - Q_i] \cdot \boldsymbol{n_i} = 0, \tag{2}$$

$$P_0 \cdot \boldsymbol{n_i} + S_x x_1 \underbrace{\boldsymbol{U} \cdot \boldsymbol{n_i}}_{\alpha_i} + S_y y_1 \underbrace{\boldsymbol{V} \cdot \boldsymbol{n_i}}_{\beta_i} = \underbrace{Q_i^t \cdot \boldsymbol{n_i}}_{d_i}, \tag{3}$$

Now assume another point (x_2, y_2) in the image that is also on the intersection line of the same phantom plane.

$$P_0 \cdot \boldsymbol{n_i} + S_x x_2 \boldsymbol{U} \cdot \boldsymbol{n_i} + S_y y_2 \boldsymbol{V} \cdot \boldsymbol{n_i} = Q_i^t \cdot \boldsymbol{n_i}, \tag{4}$$

Now by subtracting Eq. 4 from Eq. 3 and then dividing by S_x, we have:

$$\varDelta x \boldsymbol{U} \cdot \boldsymbol{n_i} + K \varDelta y \boldsymbol{V} \cdot \boldsymbol{n_i} = 0. \tag{5}$$

where $K = \frac{S_y}{S_x}$, $\varDelta x = x_2 - x_1$ and $\varDelta y = y_2 - y_1$. By dividing Eq. 5 by $\varDelta x$ and assuming $m = \frac{\varDelta y}{\varDelta x}$, we have:

$$\boldsymbol{U} \cdot \boldsymbol{n} + K m \boldsymbol{V} \cdot \boldsymbol{n} = 0. \tag{6}$$

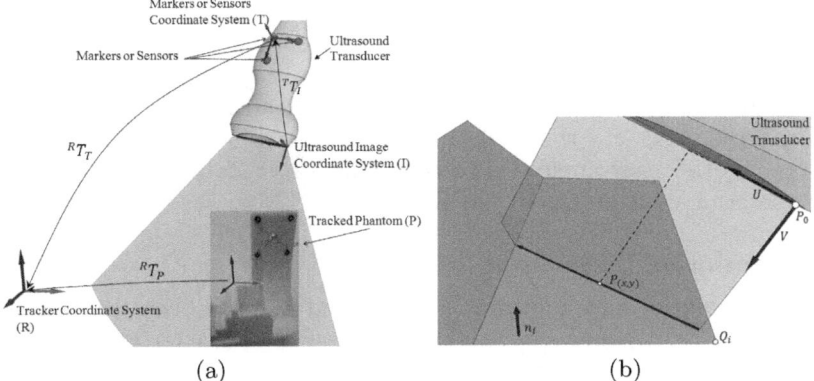

(a)   (b)

Fig. 2. (a) The coordinate system of the phantom and the ultrasound transducer. (b) Intersection of the ultrasound image and the phantom i^{th} plane .

In fact, m is the slope of the intersection line that can be measured from the ultrasound image. At least five linear equations such as Eq. 6 for five independent planes are needed to solve for the unknowns subject to the unity constraint of U and V. One can write equations in matrix form as follows:

$$N_{p\times 3}U + KM_{p\times p}N_{p\times 3}V = 0. \tag{7}$$

where $N = (n_1^t, n_2^t, \ldots, n_p^t)_{p\times 3}$, $M = diag(m_1, m_2, \ldots, m_p)_{p\times p}$ and p is the number of planes. Eq. 7 can be re-written as below:

$$\begin{bmatrix} N_{p\times 3} & MN_{p\times 3} \end{bmatrix} \begin{bmatrix} U \\ KV \end{bmatrix} = 0. \tag{8}$$

In fact, Eq. 8 is a set of linear equations with the right side equal to zero. If we divide both sides by U_x and move $-n_{i_x}$ to the right (for each row i) and define new unknowns as $X = \begin{bmatrix} \frac{u_y}{u_x} & \frac{u_z}{u_x} & K\frac{v_x}{u_x} & K\frac{v_y}{u_x} & K\frac{v_z}{u_x} \end{bmatrix}^t$, we get a set of linear equations with non-zero values on the right side:

$$\begin{bmatrix} n_{1_y} & n_{1_y} & m_1 n_{1_x} & m_1 n_{1_y} & m_1 n_{1_z} \\ \vdots & \vdots & \vdots & \vdots & \vdots \\ n_{p_y} & n_{p_y} & m_p n_{p_x} & m_p n_{p_y} & m_p n_{p_z} \end{bmatrix}_{p\times 5} \begin{bmatrix} \frac{u_y}{u_x} \\ \frac{u_z}{u_x} \\ K\frac{v_x}{u_x} \\ K\frac{v_y}{u_x} \\ K\frac{v_z}{u_x} \end{bmatrix}_{5\times 1} = -\begin{bmatrix} n_{1_x} \\ \vdots \\ n_{p_y} \end{bmatrix}_{p\times 1} \tag{9}$$

This gives a unique solution for $p = 5$ simply by solving a set of five linear equations with five unknowns (X). Then U, V and K can be uniquely found from:

$$U = \frac{[1, x_1, x_2]}{\|[1, x_1, x_2]\|}, \quad V = \frac{[x_3, x_4, x_5]}{\|[x_3, x_4, x_5]\|}, \quad K = \|[x_3, x_4, x_5]\| u_x. \tag{10}$$

This solution is the same as the Null space of Eq. 8. For $p > 5$ we can find the solution in a least-squares sense. The above derivation also explains the need for five planes. Another way of getting a non-zero value on the right side is by taking the differences of two columns on two different parallel wedges with a specified height difference. Therefore this known height difference would appear on the right side of Eq. 5. In the case of steered ultrasound beam, U and V are not orthogonal and the deviation of their crossing angle from $90°$ can be expressed as the skew angle. Up to this point, the rotational matrix, skew and S_y are determined from U, V and K.

2.3   Translation Parameters

In Eq. 3, d_i and S_x are known and S_y, U and V have been determined from previous step, so α_i and β_i are also known. For any arbitrary column x_i in the image, the position of the line y_i should be measured. Using Eq. 3 for at least three planes gives a set of linear equations with three unknowns (i.e. the coordinates of P_0) that is straight forward to solve. It can also be solved with more than three points in a least-squares sense to improve accuracy.

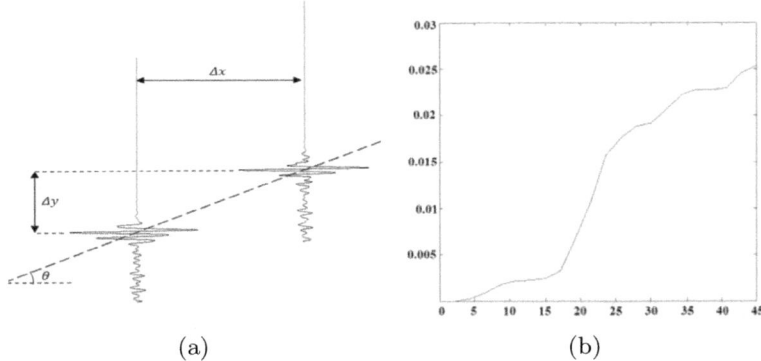

(a)   (b)

Fig. 3. (a) (Left) Slope measurement with RF cross-correlation. $\tan(\theta) = \frac{\Delta y}{\Delta x}$ (b) (Right) Slope measurement error ($\frac{Error(\Delta y)}{\Delta x}$) versus the angle between the beam and plane normal vector (φ).

2.4   Phantom Design

As mentioned, phantom design was optimized using simulated RF images from the Field II ultrasound simulation package. The goal is to find a suitable angle of each wedge so that the line segments are clear in the image and can be segmented accurately while the slopes are still large enough to achieve lowest sensitivity of the calibration results to the measurement error.

This design trade off can be better understood by explaining the RF image formation and the measurement process. Each column of an ultrasound image is formed by envelope detection of an RF echo signal. The spacing between the columns depends on the spacing of the transducer's elements, which is generally provided by the manufacturer. Axial resolution depends on the RF center frequency, the sampling rate of ultrasound machine, and speed of sound.

When imaging a flat surface with ultrasound, the RF echo pulse in each column is reflected at a specific point. All these points reside on a straight line with measurable slope (Fig. 3a). As long as the pulse shapes of at least two columns are similar, accurate slope measurement is possible by finding their axial shift with a cross correlation technique [9]. Due to the high axial resolution, a very accurate measurement can be performed. If the ultrasound beam axis is perpendicular to the surface, the shape of the RF pulses in all the columns will be the same since they all experience the same physical conditions. However, the shape of the returned echo changes slightly as the angle between the beam axis and the normal of the surface increases. This is because of the non-uniform point spread function of the ultrasound beam.

In the Field II simulation package, we modeled a plane with a number of discrete scatterers. The angle between the beam axis and the plane normal, φ, is chosen in the interval of 0 to 30 degrees and the error in the slope measurement is calculated (Fig. 3b). Results show that as the plane tilts towards higher angles with respect to the ultrasound beam, the change in the pulse shape for different columns leads to larger errors in slope measurement. These results agree with our experimental results when imaging a flat metallic surface immersed in water in different poses. In this work, the phantom is constructed with $10°$ wedges as a reasonable compromise.

3   Results

3.1   Calibration Repeatability

For calibration, 15 different images of the multi-wedge phantom are acquired. All the images are processed in a semi-automatic procedure where the user verifies the suggested line segments found by a line detection algorithm and, if necessary, identifies the appropriate edge points of each line segment. Then based on the cross correlation technique, the slope of each line is calculated from pairs of RF data. Lastly, after fitting a line to each segment, the middle point (x_i) is taken and its depth (y_i) is automatically measured from the peak of the RF pulse. Although this value is an absolute measurement, with greater inherent error than differential measurements, the result (translation parameters) is not very sensitive to this measurement (investigated later in this section). To evaluate the calibration repeatability, the calibration is solved using all the images except one for all 15 possible combinations and the standard deviation is calculated (Table. 1). Similarly, the calibration is evaluated using different numbers (n_s) of images. Each time, $n_s(=2$ to $14)$ images are randomly chosen from all 15 images and the calibration is solved. The standard deviation and the average of the results over 250 iterations have been calculated and shown in Fig. 4. It shows that standard deviation of error rapidly decreases as the number of input images increases and a few number of images are sufficient to achieve very accurate results. Note that given the closed-form formulation, the order of the images is unimportant.

3.2   Calibration Accuracy

In order to evaluate the calibration results, an independent validation experiment was performed. A set of six independent wires similar to a double N-wire phantom in [7] was integrated into the phantom (Fig. 1). The position of the wires is measured by a tracked stylus. 50 different images of this N-wire phantom were then acquired from different transducer positions. Using the calculated calibration matrix, and the measurements of the poses of the transducer and the

Table 1. Standard deviation of 15 calibration results using 14 images at a time

	Rotaion ($°$)			Translation(mm)		
	r_x	r_y	r_z	t_x	t_y	t_z
Error Standard Deviation	0.005	0.18	0.37	0.02	0.02	0.18

Table 2. Calibration accuracy in terms of point reconstruction error (300 points)

Error	Standard deviation (mm)	Mean(mm)
x	0.22	0.25
y	0.12	0.11
Distance	0.23	0.29

wires from the tracker, the six intersection points of the wires with the ultrasound image were estimated in ultrasound image coordinates. These estimated points were then compared to the actual points appearing in the image. The centroid of these points were also segmented manually and the error in x and y directions and the Euclidian distance error are calculated for all points ($50 \times 6 = 300$) and shown in Table. 2.

3.3 Sensitivity to Absolute Measurement

As mentioned, skew, scale and rotation parameters are calculated using accurate differential measurements, but to find translation parameters, absolute depth (y_i) of the lines at column x_i is measured from the peak of the RF pulse.

Therefore we can assume there is an error in measurement of y_i which can be modeled as a random noise in the range of the pulse length (0.1 mm). To evaluate the sensitivity of calibration translation parameters to this error, a random noise

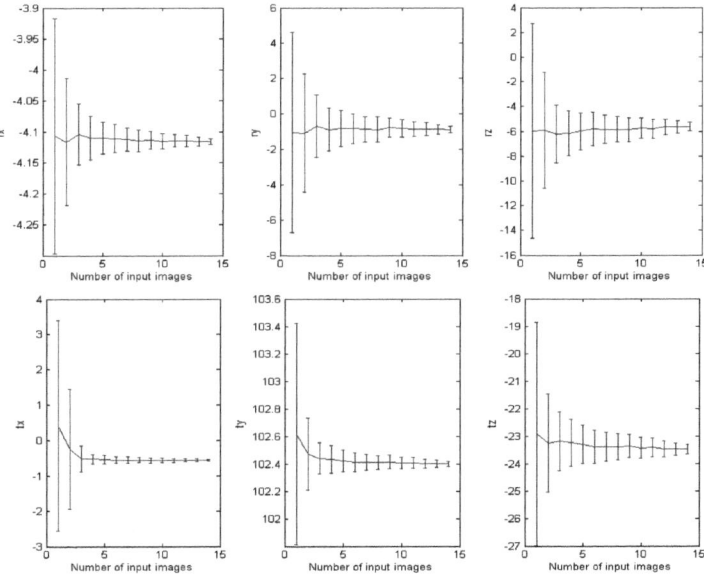

Fig. 4. Calibration results using 2 to 14 images of the phantom (top) Translation parameters (t_x, t_y, t_z) [mm] (bottom) Rotation parameters (r_x, r_y, r_z) [deg]

Table 3. STD of error in the translation parameters when normal noise ($\sigma = 0.1\ mm$) added to y_i

STD of error in translation parameters(mm)		
x	y	z
0.19	0.02	0.2

having a normal distribution ($\sigma = 0.1\ mm$) has been added to y_i measurements and the standard deviation of the translation parameters have been calculated (1000 iterations) and shown in Table. 3. Note that the true surface (wedge) location is not necessarily the peak of the RF pulse and is not easy to find [10], but the true surface lies within the echo, so any remaining systematic errors should be less than the pulse length.

4   Discussion and Conclusion

In this paper, a novel closed-form method is proposed for freehand $3D$ ultrasound calibration that extends upon previous calibration techniques. The method has been developed based on the specific physical properties of ultrasound imaging system. The relative shift of two RF-echo pulses hitting the same plane surface seems to be a very accurate measure to base a calibration technique. With this in mind, based on the simulations and the experiments, a multi-wedge phantom has been proposed. There is a trade-off in the design of the phantom. For a given measurement error the calibration error decreases as the surfaces in the phantom become steeper and more distanced from each other but on the other hand, the measurement error for those surfaces gets larger.

Experimental results show that a few (~ 10) images of the phantom are required for high accuracy. Also, independent accuracy evaluation of the calibration results confirms the high accuracy of the proposed method. Location of target points (N-wire intersections with the ultrasound imaging plane) has been estimated with less than 0.3 mm accuracy. This accuracy also includes the error from segmentation of the points, so calibration error is less than this total.

Although it is incorrect to compare calibration accuracy between systems with different transducers, ultrasound machines, and trackers, it is worth citing an example where 10,000 images of the double N-wire phantom gave a point reconstruction error of 0.66 mm [7]. The authors could not find previous calibration results with an accuracy of 0.3 mm.

The phantom can be enclosed in a sterile fluid-filled rubber-topped box for intra-operative use. The calibration procedure is very easy and fast by taking several images of the phantom in a fast sweep. Image processing can be performed in real-time. Therefore, calibration will take less than one minute.

Future work will extend this method to curvilinear and 3D transducers. Our initial investigations show that a new formulation based on polar coordinates requires even fewer numbers of images because many more plane orientations are available in a single image due to the non-parallel nature of the beams.

Such work will proceed on both pre- and post-scan converted data. Given the inexpensive and easy manufacturing of the phantom, this calibration method can be disseminated to a wide range of researchers by sharing CAD files and program code.We will integrate the software in the PLUS library for public use.

Acknowledgments. This work is supported by the Natural Sciences and Engineering Research Council of Canada (NSERC) and Canadian Institutes of Health Research (CIHR).

References

1. Lindseth, F., Lang, T., Bang, J., Nagelhus Hernes, T.A.: Accuracy evaluation of a 3D ultrasound-based neuronavigation system. Computer Aided Surgery: Official Journal of the International Society for Computer Aided Surgery 7(4), 197–222 (2002); PMID: 12454892
2. Gulati, S., Berntsen, E.M., Solheim, O., Kvistad, K.A., Hberg, A., Selbekk, T., Torp, S.H., Unsgaard, G.: Surgical resection of high-grade gliomas in eloquent regions guided by blood oxygenation level dependent functional magnetic resonance imaging, diffusion tensor tractography, and intraoperative navigated 3D ultrasound. Minimally Invasive Neurosurgery: MIN 52(1), 17–24 (2009); PMID: 19247900
3. Mercier, L., Lang, T., Lindseth, F., Collins, D.L.: A review of calibration techniques for freehand 3-D ultrasound systems. Ultrasound in Medicine & Biology 31(4), 449–471 (2005); PMID: 15831324
4. Hsu, P., Prager, R., Gee, A., Treece, G., Sensen, C., Hallgrmsson, B.: Freehand 3D ultrasound calibration: A review. Advanced Imaging in Biology and Medicine, 47–84 (2009)
5. Prager, R.W., Rohling, R.N., Gee, A.H., Berman, L.: Rapid calibration for 3-D freehand ultrasound. Ultrasound in Medicine & Biology 24(6), 855–869 (1998)
6. Boctor, E.M., Iordachita, I., Choti, M.A., Hager, G., Fichtinger, G.: Bootstrapped ultrasound calibration. Studies in Health Technology and Informatics 119, 61–66 (2006); PMID: 16404015
7. Chen, T.K., Thurston, A.D., Ellis, R.E., Abolmaesumi, P.: A Real-Time freehand ultrasound calibration system with automatic accuracy feedback and control. Ultrasound in Medicine & Biology 35(1), 79–93 (2009)
8. Afsham, N., Chan, K., Pan, L., Tang, S., Rohling, R.N.: Alignment and calibration of high frequency ultrasound (HFUS) and optical coherence tomography (OCT) 1D transducers using a dual wedge-tri step phantom. In: Proceedings of SPIE, vol. 7964, p. 796428 (March 2011)
9. Zahiri-Azar, R., Salcudean, S.E.: Motion estimation in ultrasound images using time domain cross correlation with prior estimates. IEEE Transactions on Biomedical Engineering 53(10), 1990–2000 (2006)
10. Hacihaliloglu, I., Abugharbieh, R., Hodgson, A.J., Rohling, R.N.: Bone surface localization in ultrasound using image Phase-Based features. Ultrasound in Medicine & Biology 35, 1475–1487 (2009)

Model-Based Respiratory Motion Compensation in MRgHIFU

Patrik Arnold[1], Frank Preiswerk[1], Beat Fasel[1], Rares Salomir[2], Klaus Scheffler[3], and Philippe Cattin[1]

[1] Medical Image Analysis Center, University of Basel, Switzerland
patrik.arnold@unibas.ch
[2] Radiology Department, University Hospitals of Geneva, Switzerland
[3] Department of Neuroimaging, University of Tuebingen, Germany

Abstract. Magnetic Resonance guided High Intensity Focused Ultrasound (MRgHIFU) is an emerging non-invasive technology for the treatment of pathological tissue. The possibility of depositing sharply localised energy deep within the body without affecting the surrounding tissue requires the exact knowledge of the target's position. The cyclic respiratory organ motion renders targeting challenging, as the treatment focus has to be continuously adapted according to the current target's displacement in 3D space. In this paper, a combination of a patient-specific dynamic breath model and a population-based statistical motion model is used to compensate for the respiratory induced organ motion. The application of a population based statistical motion model replaces the acquisition of a patient-specific 3D motion model, nevertheless allowing for precise motion compensation.

1 Introduction

Focused Ultrasound deposits sharply localised energy in the tissue causing thermal ablation. Precise targeting demands for exact knowledge of the target's position. The compensation of the fitful respiratory organ motion is a challenging task in the treatment of pathological tissue in abdominal organs. If breathing motion is not compensated, the exposure of healthy tissue increases and the thermal dose delivered to the tumour is reduced. Continuous target displacement tracking in 3D space requires accurate spatial and rapid temporal beam refocusing in the range of millimetres and milliseconds, respectively. Any realisation of a real-time target tracking-based dose delivery must thus be able to predict the target's position at some future time in order to compensate for the finite time delay between the acquisition of the current target's position and the mechanical response of the system to change treatment focus.

During sonication the Magnetic Resonance (MR) scan-time is mainly required for the temperature feedback control of the High Intensity Focused Ultrasound (HIFU) system, quantifying the thermal dose given to the tissue in order to guarantee complete coagulation of the tumour. Therefore, not enough MR scan-time is left to track the tumour in 3D. To determine the thermal dose, temperature maps in regular distances around the tumour are acquired. Similarly as proposed in [1], the navigator (pencil beam) feedback information is used to reposition the temperature mapping slice to resolve organ

P. Abolmaesumi et al. (Eds.): IPCAI 2012, LNAI 7330, pp. 54–63, 2012.

displacements. In this work, we propose to use this 1-dimensional navigator feedback information not only to track the current respiratory state, but also to predict the organ's future displacement, e.g. the position of the tumour.

Several approaches have been proposed to track and predict the motion of abdominal organs. Ries *et al.* [1] proposed a real-time tracking method that observes the target on a 2D image plane combined with a perpendicular acquired pencil beam navigator, providing quasi-3D information of the target trajectories. The future 3D target position is then estimated by a Kalman filter. Underlying a regular and stable breathing pattern, the method was tested in phantom experiments and in vivo on ventilated pigs. The accuracy of the approach is not evaluated on ground truth motion data, but by indirectly comparing the temperature maps obtained after 60 seconds of HIFU sonication with and without motion compensation, resulting in higher maximal temperatures in the target area with enabled motion compensation. However, the experiments have neither been evaluated on ground truth data nor under free breathing conditions.

Ruan and Keall [2] proposed a predictor based on Kernel Density Estimation to account for system latencies caused by software and hardware processing. They use 3D motion trajectories of implanted markers to train the predictor in a lower dimensional feature space using Principal Component Analysis (PCA). The prediction is performed in this subspace and mapped back into the original space for the evaluation. The drawback of the method is that only the position of directly observed internal fiducials can be predicted and not of the entire organ.

Only recently, a combination of a pattern matching approach using a static subject-specific model and a population-based statistical drift model for motion-compensated MRgHIFU treatment was described and evaluated on realistic 4DMRI data [3]. While the results are convincing, the acquisition of a patient-specific 3D motion atlas takes several minutes and the processing time is in the range of hours and thus is not acceptable for clinical use. In particular, the multiple volume-to-volume registrations take up to several hours, in which the patient is asked not to move in order to stay aligned with the acquired model.

Preiswerk *et al.* [4] showed, that the displacement of the entire liver can be spatially predicted by tracking three well distributed markers (implanted fiducials) within the liver using a population-based statistical motion model. Based on an exhalation breath-hold scan, accurate prediction is achieved. Dispensing with the need of extensive pretreatment volume imaging and its time consuming 3D non-rigid registration, no attention is payed to a potential system lag, which is essential for real-time tracking. Also this method is based on full 3D motion information of implanted markers.

The main contribution of the presented work is the combination of a patient-specific fast and lightweight respiratory breathing model and a population-based motion model to a novel, completely non-invasive and clinically feasible 3D motion compensation method for MRgHIFU treatments. The proposed method addresses certain weaknesses of the state-of-the-art methods in terms of real-time usage and validation. On the one hand, the completely MR-based respiratory signal is continuously acquired and used to predict the organs future respiratory state in order to bridge the system's time delay between the tracking and treatment of the target. On the other hand, the population-based motion model is applied to estimate the motion of the unobserved liver, without the need of acquiring a subject-specific 3D motion model.

2   Materials and Methods

For the evaluation of our approach, a realistic MRgHIFU scenario was assumed. During HIFU sonication, the measured information of the pencil beam navigator, *i.e.* the inferior-superior displacement (1D) of the diaphragm, is used as the *breathing signal*. Based on this *breathing signal* a patient-specific respiratory model is created, whereby a temporal prediction of the diaphragm's future position is estimated (Sec. 2.2). Having an estimate of this displacement, the population-based statistical model is used to compute the most likely 3D displacement of the entire liver, further referred as to *reconstruction* (Sec. 2.3).

2.1   Data and Ground Truth

The ground truth data was acquired by 4DMRI, a dynamic 2D MR imaging method capturing the respiratory motion during free breathing [5]. Thanks to the sagittal slice orientation and the interleaved acquisition of data slices and a dedicated so-called *navigator slice* at a fixed position, vascular structures used for the 3D reconstruction of the volumes are visible during complete breathing cycles and can be tracked with minimal out-of-plane motion. 4DMRI sequences of 20 healthy volunteers (mixed sexes, age range: 17-75) were captured. During acquisition sessions of roughly two hours, 20-45 minutes of time-resolved organ motion data was measured. MR volumes consisting of 25-30 slices (120×192 pixel) covering the right liver lobe with a voxel size of $1.4 \times 1.4 \times 4$ mm^3 and with a temporal resolution of 300-400 ms were obtained. The retrospectively reconstructed 3D stacks cover the entire range of observed breathing depths. By means of B-spline-based 3D non-rigid registration [6], dense spatio-temporal vector fields describing the motion between the different respiratory states of the liver are extracted. The first manually segmented liver exhalation stack is taken as reference volume upon which the subsequent 3D stacks are incrementally registered from time-step to time-step. The vector field from the previous step is taken as an initial estimation, significantly speeding up the registration time and making the registration more robust by reducing the chance of getting trapped in a local minima. The resulting vector fields, describing the liver's displacements relative to the reference volume, serve as the basic data for the motion model and its evaluation in cross-validation experiments.

In order to build a statistical model from this data, inter-subject correspondence had to be established. For each subject mechanical corresponding points were manually selected on the reference volume surfaces in order to align the 20 datasets. These points mark the delineations between the superior surface in contact with lung, the anterior and the posterior areas, which slide along the abdominal wall, and the inferior surface. An isotropic grid with 10 mm resolution was placed in the resulting average liver and then transformed to the shape of each of the subjects. This finally gave a set of 20 topologically equivalent 3D liver volumes as well as vector fields describing the motion

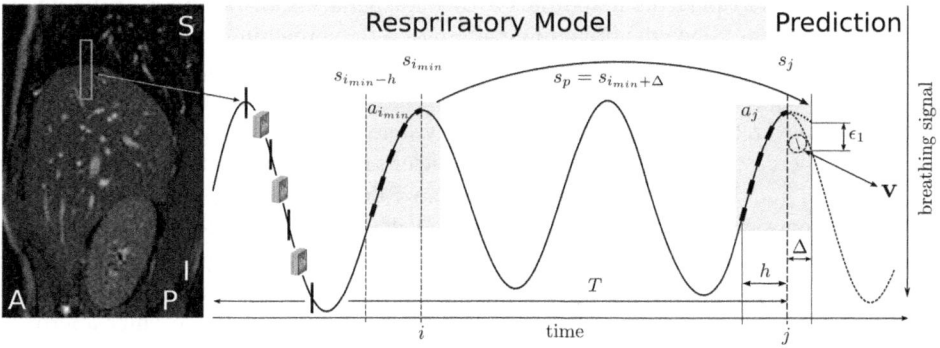

Fig. 1. Schematic illustration of combined respiratory model and motion model-based prediction. Based on the respiratory signal (|) captured at the marked diaphragm region, the displacement s_p of the diaphragm is predicted and from that the full liver displacement $\mathbf{v}$ is *reconstructed*.

for each of the $N = 1261$ inter-subject corresponding grid points. For more detailed information we refer the reader to the article of Preiswerk *et al.* [4].

In this work, the described *breathing signal* is generated by simulating a pencil beam navigator placed on the acquired *navigator slices*. A manually defined region placed anywhere at the diaphragm was persistently tracked by template matching (Normalised Cross Correlation) throughout the acquisition sequence providing one respiratory position and displacement per acquired *navigator slice*, respectively. The inferior-superior component of the templates motion is interpreted as the *breathing signal* as obtained by a common pencil beam navigator, see Figures 1 and 2(a). The spatial resolution is thus given by the image's pixel size of roughly $1.4 \times 1.4\,\mathrm{mm}^2$.

Since the 3D volumes are reconstructed at the time point between two *navigator slices* (see Figure 1, *left*) we linearly interpolate the *breathing signal* in order to obtain the respiratory positions and the 3D volumes at the same time points for the evaluation. In the following we deal with a linearly interpolated *breathing signal* with a sample rate of 6-8 Hz.

2.2 Temporal Prediction

Figure 1 schematically illustrates the prediction scene for the combined patient-specific and population-based model. As described above, the *breathing signal* is extracted by tracking a defined region on all the *navigator slices* followed by linear interpolation obtaining the intermediate respiratory states, where the ground truth 3D data is available for the validation.

The temporal prediction of the *breathing signal* is necessary in order to compensate for the system lag, caused by the pencil beam acquisition time, the processing of the data and the time for refocusing the HIFU beam to the newly calculated target. Any breathing-controlled tracking method must thus be able to estimate the target's position at some future time. The prediction of the future curve of the *breathing signal* is a key part of the prediction pipeline. Faulty predictions lead to wrong assumptions on the diaphragm's displacement and thus to wrong spatial *reconstructions* of the whole liver displacement. Since the breathing pattern of a free breathing patient is very irregular over time, e.g. the amplitude and phase are changing nearly unpredictably, we use a prediction algorithm which can quickly adapt to the new input data. In the proposed method, however, the tracking of the respiratory state during sonication is based on pencil beams, therefore, one can expect a much lower sampling rate, as for example given by an optical tracking system. In our simulation we deal with a sampling rate of 6-8 Hz. Due to the low sampling rate, the learning based algorithms would lead to considerable prediction errors at each ex- and inhalation position before adapting. Therefore we use a similar technique as proposed in [3], where a one-dimensional breathing model based on the measured pencil beam navigators is created. In contrast to the latter approach where the model is acquired in a training phase and then stays fixed, our respiratory model steadily grows even during increasing treatment time T. Each newly measured data point (pencil beam position) is added to the model, thus getting more and more stable over time. As the prediction algorithm prefers the most recent measurements in the model, the model can be kept small to avoid a system slowdown caused by the increasing model size. All the data stored in the model is observed for the patient-specific operational setup, therefore only realistic displacements of the liver are predicted. For anomalous breathing patterns with a deviation from the breath model above a certain threshold, *i.e.* no matching pattern is found (*e.g.* coughing, new pattern), the HIFU beam can be switched off to ensure patient safety.

The model is best represented by a matrix $\mathbf{A}$, wherein the *breathing signal* is piecewise stored:

$$\mathbf{A} = \begin{pmatrix} s_1 & s_2 & \cdots & s_h & s_{h+\Delta} \\ s_2 & s_3 & \cdots & s_{h+1} & s_{h+1+\Delta} \\ \vdots & \vdots & & \vdots & \vdots \\ s_{i-h} & s_{i-h+1} & \cdots & s_i & s_{i+\Delta} \\ \vdots & \vdots & & \vdots & \vdots \\ s_{T-h} & s_{T-h+1} & \cdots & s_T & s_{T+\Delta} \end{pmatrix}. \tag{1}$$

The temporal prediction is based on the last h values of the current *breathing signal* given by the vector $\mathbf{a}_j = (s_{j-h}, \ldots, s_j)$, where the index j denotes the actual time point. The prediction provides an estimate $s_p = s'_{j+\Delta}$ describing the future signal curve for a later time point, Δ time steps ahead. The best matching pattern of the current *breathing signal* vector $\mathbf{a}_j$ and the column vectors $\mathbf{a}_i$ of $\mathbf{A}$, is found with:

$$i_{min} = \arg \min_i \{|\mathbf{a}_i - \mathbf{a}_j|, |j - T|\}. \tag{2}$$

The future curve of $\mathbf{a}_{i_{min}}$ with minimum aberration from the actual signal's history $\mathbf{a}_j$ is considered as best estimate of the organ's future respiratory state:

$$s_p = s_{i_{min}+\Delta}. \tag{3}$$

The resulting prediction error ϵ_1 is then given by:

$$\epsilon_1 = |s_{j+\Delta} - s_p|. \tag{4}$$

The value s_p is the predicted shift in inferior-superior direction of the next diaphragm position. This displacement serves as the input to the motion model that then predicts the position of the entire liver. As the algorithm is continuously adjusting to new input data and updated with the new measured signal input, it can quickly adapt to the irregularity of the periods and amplitudes of the respiratory signal of a free breathing person. Figure 2(b) shows 60 seconds of robust 170 ms ahead prediction performance of an irregular breathing pattern measured by template matching (*blue*) and the model-based prediction (*green*) of subject 4.

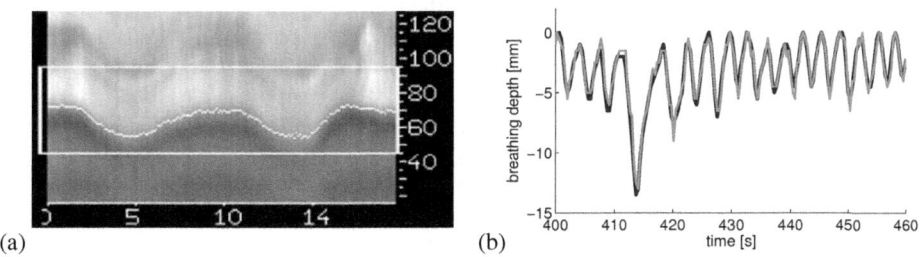

(a)   (b)

Fig. 2. (a) Typical pencil-beam navigator for MR thermometry real-time slice correction acquired at 10 Hz. (b) Example of 170 ms ahead prediction of a irregular breathing pattern of subject 4. Blue: tracked *breathing signal*; Green: robust respiratory model-based prediction.

2.3 Statistical Modelling

So far, the displacement of only one single point at the diaphragm is known from the prediction. The observed region, the centre of the pencil beam navigator template located on the *navigator slice*, respectively, has to be adopted to the closest grid-point of the subject's liver. The predicted shift s_p is then rigidly assigned to the corresponding model grid-point and the population-based statistical model is used for the *reconstruction* of the entire non-rigid liver displacement. From each of the 20 subjects, the vector fields of the first 15 breathing cycles are taken to build the model. The liver displacements are represented by a $3N$-dimensional vector $\mathbf{v} = (\Delta u_1, \Delta v_1, \Delta w_1, \ldots, \Delta u_N, \Delta v_N, \Delta w_N)'$. Note, that the difference vector $\mathbf{v}$ contains no shape information, but only the relative displacements with respect to the reference volume. The vector fields are mean-free concatenated in a data matrix $\mathbf{X} = (\mathbf{x}_1, \mathbf{x}_2, \ldots, \mathbf{x}_m) \in \mathbb{R}^{3N \times m}$ with $\mathbf{x}_k = \mathbf{v}_k - \bar{\mathbf{v}}$ and sample mean $\bar{\mathbf{v}} = \frac{1}{m} \sum_{k=1}^{m} \mathbf{v}_k$. Applying PCA to the data, the vectors $\mathbf{x}$ are defined by the coefficients c_k and the Eigenvectors $\mathbf{s}_k$ of $\mathbf{S} = (\mathbf{s}_1, \mathbf{s}_2, \ldots)$ of the covariance matrix of the data:

$$\mathbf{x} = \sum_{k=1}^{m-1} c_k \sigma_k \mathbf{s}_k = \mathbf{S} \cdot \mathrm{diag}(\sigma_k)\, \mathbf{c}\,. \tag{5}$$

Hereby, $\sigma_\mathbf{k}$ are the standard deviations within the data along each eigenvector s_k . As elaborated in [7], the model coefficient $\mathbf{c}$ for the full vector $\mathbf{x}$ can be found by an incomplete estimate $s_p \in \mathbb{R}^l, l < N$ that minimises

$$E(\mathbf{c}) = ||\mathbf{Qc} - s_p|| + \eta \cdot ||\mathbf{c}||^2\,, \tag{6}$$

with $\mathbf{Q} = \mathbf{LS} \cdot \mathrm{diag}(\sigma_k)$, where $\mathbf{L}$ represents a subspace mapping $\mathbf{L} : \mathbb{R}^N \mapsto \mathbb{R}^l$. In the case of a noisy or incorrect assumption s_p, tuning the regularisation factor η allows for *reconstructions* closer to the average quantified by the Mahalanobis distance $||\mathbf{c}||^2$. Solving Eq. 6 for $\mathbf{c}$ with the singular value decomposition of $\mathbf{Q} = \overline{\mathbf{V}}\mathbf{W}\mathbf{V}^T$, yields:

$$\mathbf{c} = \mathbf{V}\,\mathrm{diag}(\frac{w_k}{w_k^2 + \eta})\,\overline{\mathbf{V}}^T s_p\,. \tag{7}$$

Using Eq. 7 the most probable organ displacement under the constraint of the known one-dimensional point-shift prediction s_p is then given by:

$$\mathbf{v} = \mathbf{S} \cdot \mathrm{diag}(\sigma_k)\,\mathbf{c} + \bar{\mathbf{v}}\,. \tag{8}$$

The elaborated framework allows to associate the rigid 1D shift of 1 point placed at the diaphragm with the non-rigid 3D motion of the entire liver based on population statistics.

3   Experiments and Results

To evaluate the prediction performance of the algorithm for clinical relevant motion compensation, experiments on 20 volunteer subjects were performed. On average, displacements of the diaphragm from 5.5 mm to 15.2 mm in inferior-superior direction depending on the subject were observed. For simplicity of generating population statistics, the same amount of data from each subject was included for the experiments. For each experiment 1500 time steps, corresponding to 7-11 minutes, have been predicted.

In a first step, the prediction performance of the respiratory model is tested and evaluated on each of the subjects. In a second step, the respiratory model and the motion model prediction are evaluated in combination with cross-validation experiments. The predictive scene was evaluated every 300-400 ms, at the time points where the ground truth 3D data is available. All experiments were performed with a lookahead length of $\Delta = 1$, *i.e.* 150-200 ms and based on a signal history length of $h = 4$, corresponding to roughly 0.7 s.

3.1   Breath Prediction

Theoretically, the algorithm is able to predict after the first $h = 4$ time steps (≈ 0.7 s). But as more breathing cycles are collected in the respiratory model the more robust the method is predicting. Therefore, we observed the behavior of predictive performance as a function of time, *i.e.* with an increasing model size. Figure 3(a) shows the average error cumulated up to the given time on the axis and error bars showing the standard deviation. The error in prediction is retrospectively computed according to Eq.(4).

In Figure 3(b) the overall results of breath prediction for all 20 subject are visualised by error bars, marking the average and standard deviations. The experiments are evaluated after a model acquisition time of 60 seconds. The average error over all subjects is 0.6 mm with an observed average breathing depth of 8.4 mm.

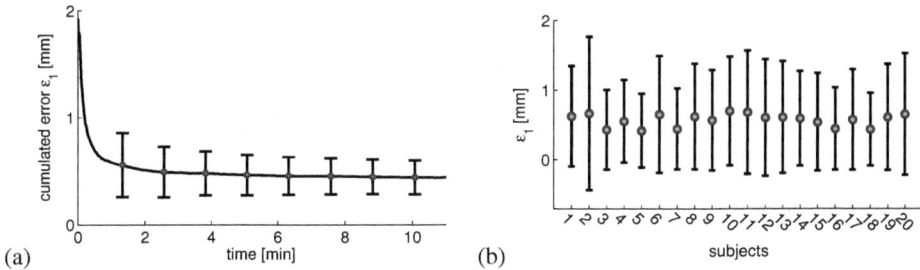

(a)   (b)

Fig. 3. (a) Average and standard deviations of the cumulated breath prediction error averaged over all subjects. The performance stabilises after a few minutes and is acceptable after 60 seconds. (b) Prediction performance of the respiratory model evaluated for 20 subjects averaged over a prediction length of 7-11 minutes, whereby the first 60 seconds are used to acquire a minimal model. The results are presented by error bars, marking the average and standard deviations for lookahead time of $\Delta_t \approx 180$ ms and signal history length of $h_t \approx 0.7$ s with an overall error of 0.6 mm.

3.2 Motion Model Prediction

The minimum size of population data to create a reliable model is still a unsolved problem as the exact distribution of the data for the entire population is unknown. The suitability of statistical models can, however, be shown empirically in cross-validation experiments. For the evaluation of our motion prediction technique leave-one-out statistical models of all the 20 subjects were computed. From the left-out data a respiratory signal was generated and used as test signal. As explained in Section 2.2 and 2.3, the respiratory motion of the full liver is predicted from one single point at the diaphragm only. For the *reconstruction* we took the 9 first principal components ending up with a model covering 98% of the variance of the original motion data. For each subject the manual segmentation of a reference volume and establishing correspondence (Sec. 2.1) is necessary.

As the predicted shift s_p can not fully be accounted for, the regularisation factor of Eq. (7) was set to $\eta = 5.5$ in order to get more plausible *reconstructions*. The error of prediction is determined by the point-wise Euclidean distance from the predicted liver motion to the ground truth motion of the left-out liver. To give an overview of the error distribution the results are visualised in Figure 4(a) by the median and error bars marking the 25th and 75th percentiles. The dashed line is set to 2 mm, marking an acceptable accuracy limit for HIFU treatments [8]. The average error over all subjects is 1.7 mm, in contrast to the average error without any motion compensation of 3.8 mm. In the case of no motion compensation, the error equals to the mean of the Euclidean distances to the reference volume over time. The spatial distribution of the averaged error over all subjects and time steps is shown in Figure 4(b). The root cause of the error are false predictions in inferior-superior and anterior-posterior direction with a maximal error of 2 mm, 1.1 mm and a minor error in left-right direction of 0.4 mm, respectively.

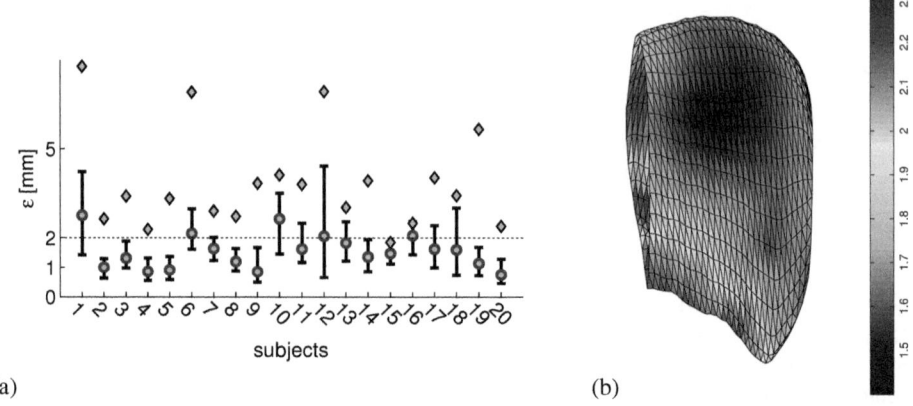

Fig. 4. (a) Resulting deviations between predicted and ground truth liver motions for 20 different subject over a time interval of 7-11 minutes. Error bars around the median show the 25th and 75th percentile deviation and mean error without any motion compensation ($\diamond$). (b) Averaged liver surface from 20 subjects of the right liver lobe at exhalation in anterior view. The colors represent the motion prediction error (in *mm*) averaged over 20 subjects at the liver's surface.

4   Conclusion

We presented a completely non-invasive and purely MR-based tracking method to predict the liver's 3D motion in real-time under free breathing. The method is a combination of a pattern matching approach to predict the patient-specific breathing pattern and a population-based statistical motion model based on PCA to *reconstruct* the respiratory induced organ motion. In the presented work, we demonstrate a safe and efficient technique for MRgHIFU treatment of pathological tissue in moving organs. Although the prediction technique is evaluated on real 4DMRI motion data of the liver, the proposed generic framework is applicable to any abdominal organ, *e.g.* the kidney. The method is evaluated on 4DMRI datasets of 20 healthy volunteers achieving an overall prediction error of 1.7 mm, where the predictive method is clinically applicable after 60 seconds.

Although the overall prediction error of our novel method is slightly higher than the state-of-the-art methods, the proposed technique addresses important issues for the non-invasive real-time application of MRgHIFU treatment in moving abdominal organs. Preiswerk *et al.* [4] achieve a prediction error of 1.2 mm by accurately knowing the 3D displacements of three well distributed points within the liver (*e.g.* implanted surrogate markers). In [3] a prediction error of 1.1 mm is achieved by acquiring 3D information of the patient specific liver motion.

In this work, however, a non-invasive MR-based tracking method is used, allowing to measure the 1-dimensional displacement of a single point on the diaphragm only. We are fully aware of that the second order organ deformation occurring over large time scales, the so called drifts, are not detectable by measuring a single point at the diaphragm only. But, since we are predicting over a short period of time, the different respiratory states of the liver can reliable be tracked, as has been shown in [9]. Besides a 3D exhalation breath-hold scan, no patient-specific 3D motion data has to be acquired and processed in a pretreatment phase.

In future work we will investigate the possibility of better adapting the population-based motion model to a specific subject. Using a fast MR acquisition sequence, we plan on better restricting the population-based statistical motion model to a specific patient.

Acknowledgments. This work has been supported by the research network of the Swiss National Science Foundation-Project Nr. CR32I3_125499.

References

1. Ries, M., de Senneville, B.D., Roujol, S., Berber, Y., Quesson, B., Moonen, C.: Real-Time 3D Target Tracking in MRI Guided Focused Ultrasound Ablations in Moving Tissues. Magnetic Resonance in Medicine 64, 1704–1712 (2010)
2. Ruan, D., Keall, P.: Online Prediction of Respiratory Motion: Multidimensional Processing with Low-Dimensional Feature Learning. Physics in Medicine and Biology 55, 3011–3025 (2010)
3. Arnold, P., Preiswerk, F., Fasel, B., Salomir, R., Scheffler, K., Cattin, P.C.: 3D Organ Motion Prediction for MR-Guided High Intensity Focused Ultrasound. In: Fichtinger, G., Martel, A., Peters, T. (eds.) MICCAI 2011, Part II. LNCS, vol. 6892, pp. 623–630. Springer, Heidelberg (2011)
4. Preiswerk, F., Arnold, P., Fasel, B., Cattin, P.C.: A Bayesian Framework for Estimating Respiratory Liver Motion from Sparse Measurements. In: Yoshida, H., Sakas, G., Linguraru, M.G. (eds.) Abdominal Imaging. LNCS, vol. 7029, pp. 207–214. Springer, Heidelberg (2012)
5. von Siebenthal, M., Szekely, G., Gamper, U., Boesiger, P., Lomax, A., Cattin, P.: 4D MR Imaging of Respiratory Organ Motion and its Variability. Phys. in Med. Biol. 52, 1547–1564 (2007)
6. Rueckert, D., Sonoda, L.I., Hayes, C., Hill, D.L.G., Leach, M.O., Hawkes, D.J.: Nonrigid Registration Using Free-Form Deformations: Application to Breast MR Images. Transactions on Medical Imaging 18, 712–721 (1999)
7. Blanz, V., Vetter, T.: Reconstructing the Complete 3D Shape of Faces from Partial Information. Informationstechnik und Technische Informatik 44, 295–302 (2002)
8. Vedam, S., Kini, V.R., Keall, P.J., Ramakrishnan, V., Mostafavi, H., Mohan, R.: Quantifying the Predictability of Diaphragm Motion During Respiration with a Noninvasive External Marker. Med. Phys. 30, 505–513 (2003)
9. von Siebenthal, M., Székely, G., Lomax, A.J., Cattin, P.C.: Systematic Errors in Respiratory Gating due to Intrafraction Deformations of the Liver. Med. Phys. 34, 3620–3629 (2007)

Non-iterative Multi-modal Partial View to Full View Image Registration Using Local Phase-Based Image Projections

Ilker Hacihaliloglu[1], David R. Wilson[1], Michael Gilbart[1], Michael Hunt[2], and
Purang Abolmaesumi[3]

[1] Departments of Orthopaedics
[2] Physical Therapy
[3] Electrical and Computer Engineering
University of British Columbia, Vancouver, BC, Canada
purang@ece.ubc.ca

Abstract. Accurate registration of patient anatomy, obtained from intra-operative ultrasound (US) and preoperative computed tomography (CT) images, is an essential step to a successful US-guided computer assisted orthopaedic surgery (CAOS). Most state-of-the-art registration methods in CAOS require either significant manual interaction from the user or are not robust to the typical US artifacts. Furthermore, one of the major stumbling blocks facing existing methods is the requirement of an optimization procedure during the registration, which is time consuming and generally breaks when the initial misalignment between the two registering data sets is large. Finally, due to the limited field of view of US imaging, obtaining scans of the full anatomy is problematic, which causes difficulties during registration. In this paper, we present a new method that registers local phase-based bone features in frequency domain using image projections calculated from three-dimensional (3D) radon transform. The method is fully automatic, non-iterative, and requires no initial alignment between the two registering datasets. We also show the method's capability in registering partial view US data to full view CT data. Experiments, carried out on a phantom and six clinical pelvis scans, show an average 0.8 mm root-mean-square registration error.

Keywords: 3D ultrasound, CT, registration, local phase, radon transform, non-iterative, phase correlation, computer assisted orthopaedic surgery.

1   Introduction

With the recent advances made in imaging technology and instrumentation, image-guided interventions have been extended to address clinical problems in various orthopaedic surgical procedures such as pedicle screw placement [1], total hip arthroplasty [2], and shoulder arthoscopy [3]. In recent years, given the concerns due to high ionizing radiation of intra-operative X-ray fluoroscopy, US imaging has been

P. Abolmaesumi et al. (Eds.): IPCAI 2012, LNAI 7330, pp. 64–73, 2012.
© Springer-Verlag Berlin Heidelberg 2012

proposed as an intra-operative imaging modality to assist with these surgical procedures. US is a real-time, inexpensive and non-ionizing imaging modality. However, US imaging has several limitations including user dependent image acquisition, limited field of view, and low signal to noise ratio (SNR). In particular to orthopaedic surgical procedures, the appearance of bone surfaces in US remains strongly influenced by the beam direction, and regions corresponding to bone boundaries appear blurry [4]. In order to alleviate some of these difficulties, pre-procedure data obtained from other imaging modalities, such as CT and MRI, have been registered with US scans. The ability to perform this registration accurately, automatically, and rapidly is critical for enabling more effective US-guided procedures in CAOS.

Since the first introduction of computer assisted surgery (CAS) a number of image registration methods have been developed. Specifically for orthopaedic surgery, due to the rigid nature of bone anatomy, surface-based registration methods have gained popularity [5]. Penney et al. [5] improved the robustness of the standard ICP by randomly perturbing the point cloud positions, which allowed the algorithm to move out of some local minima and find a minimum with lower residual error. The method was validated on a phantom femur data set where a mean target registration error (TRE) of 1.17 mm was achieved. The main drawback in that method remained the manual extraction of bone surfaces from US data. Moghari and Abolmaesumi [6] proposed a point-based registration method based on Unscented Kalman Filter (UKF). Although the method improved the registration speed, accuracy and robustness compared to standard ICP the main drawback was the extraction of bone surfaces from US images, which was done manually. Recently, Brounstein et al. [7] proposed a Gaussian Mixture Model (GMM) based surface registration algorithm, where the bone surface was extracted automatically from both modalities. The root mean square distance between the registered surfaces was reported to be 0.49 mm for phantom pelvis data and 0.63 mm for clinical pelvis data.

In order to avoid the segmentation of bone surfaces from US data, intensity-based registration methods have been developed. Brendel et al. [8] proposed a surface to volume registration method. They preprocess the CT data by segmenting only the bone surfaces that could be visible in the US using the US imaging probe orientation information. These extracted bone surfaces were then registered to the B-mode US data by maximizing the sum of the overlapping gray values of pre-processed CT bone surfaces and US data. While this method showed accurate registration results, it assumed a known probe orientation for pre-processing the CT data. This assumption may not necessarily be valid, especially for fracture reduction surgeries where the US probe needs to be realigned after a fracture reduction. Penney et al. [9] used normalized cross-correlation similarity metric to register bone probability images obtained from CT and US data sets using intensity, gradient, and US shadowing artifact information. Successful registration results were reported; however, generation of US probability images depended on segmentation information obtained from several prior data sets. Gill et al. [10] simulated US images from CT data for registering bone surfaces of the spine and achieved a registration accuracy of 1.44 mm for phantom scans and 1.25 mm for sheep cadaver scans. In a recent publication, ultrasound image simulation was performed on statistical shape models [11] where a TRE less than 3 mm was reported. In order to achieve clinically acceptable registration results this technique required accurate initial alignment of the SSM and three-dimensional (3D) US data.

Most of the previously proposed US-CT registration methods either require manual interaction for segmenting bones from US images or for initial registration to bring the two surfaces closer [5-7]. Several groups have proposed methods, based on intensity and gradient information, to automate the bone segmentation process [12]. However, due to the typical US artefacts there methods remain highly sensitive to parameters settings and have been mainly limited to 2D US data. Furthermore, one of the major stumbling blocks facing all of the proposed registration methods is the requirement of an iterative optimization procedure during the registration, which is time consuming and normally does not converge if the misalignment between the two registering data sets is large. Finally, due to the limited field of view of US imaging, obtaining scans of the full anatomy is problematic which causes difficulties during the registration.

In this paper, we present a registration method that estimates the 3D rotation and translation parameters, between the CT and US volumes, in frequency domain using local phase-based image projections. The method is fully automatic, non-iterative, and requires no initial alignment between the two datasets. We also show the method's capability in registering partial view US data to full view CT data. We validate the method on pelvic scans obtain from a phantom setup as well as six clinical scans.

2   Materials and Methods

2.1   Local Phase Based Bone Surface Extraction

Hacihaliloglu et al. [13] recently proposed a method that uses 3D local phase information to extract bone surfaces from 3D US data. The local phase information is extracted by multiplying the US volumes in frequency domain with the transfer function of 3D Log-Gabor filter (*3DLG*):

$$3DLG\,(p, \omega, \theta, \phi, \omega_0, \theta_1, \phi_i) = \exp\left(-\frac{\left(\log\left(\frac{\omega}{\omega_0}\right)\right)^2}{2\left(\log\left(\frac{\kappa}{\omega_0}\right)^2\right)}\right) \times \exp\left(-\frac{\alpha(p,\theta_1,\phi_i)^2}{2\sigma_\alpha^2}\right). \quad (1)$$

Here, κ is a scaling factor used to set the bandwidth of the filter in the radial direction, and ω_0 is the filter's center spatial frequency. To achieve constant shape-ratio filters, which are geometric scalings of the reference filter, the term κ/ω_0 must be kept constant. The angle between the direction of the filter, which is determined by the azimuth (ϕ) and elevation (θ) angles, and the position vector of a given point p in the frequency domain expressed in Cartesian coordinates in the spectral domain is given by $\alpha(p,\ \phi_i,\ \theta_i) = arcos(p \times v_i / \|p\|)$, where $v_i = (cos\phi_i \times cos\theta_i,\ cos\phi_i \times sin\theta_i, sin\phi_i)$ is a unit vector in the filter's direction and σ_α is the standard deviation of the Gaussian function in the angular direction that describes the filter's angular selectivity. To obtain higher orientation selectivity, the angular function needs to be narrower. The scaling of the radial Log-Gabor function is controlled using different wavelengths that are based on multiples of a minimum wavelength, λ_{min}, a user-defined parameter. The filter scale m, and center frequency ω_0 are related as $\omega_0 = 2/\lambda_{min} \times (\delta)^{m-1}$ where δ is a scaling factor defined for computing the center frequencies of successive filters. By using the above 3D filter over a number of scales (*m*) and at different orientations (*i*), a 3D phase symmetry (PS) measure can then defined as in (2):

$$PS_{3D}(x,y,z) = \frac{\sum_i \sum_m \lfloor [|e_{im}(x,y,z)| - |o_{im}(x,y,z)|] - T_i \rfloor}{\sum_i \sum_m \sqrt{e_{im}^2(x,y,z) + o_{im}^2(x,y,z)} + \varepsilon}. \tag{2}$$

The even and odd components, $e_{im}(x, y, z)$ and $o_{im}(x, y, z)$, of *3DLG* are calculated using the real and imaginary responses of the Log-Gabor filter for each voxel point (x, y, z). T_i is a threshold to account for noise in the US image and ε is a small number to avoid division by zero [13]. Using this method local phase bone surfaces were extracted from both US and CT data set, which are denoted as PS_{3DCT} and PS_{3DUS} from this point on. Since US imaging modality can only image the top surface of bone ray casting is applied to the local phase bone surface extracted from CT volume set leaving only the top surface of the bone that could be imaged with US. These two local phase bone surfaces are used as input to the next step.

2.2   Local Phase Projection Space from 3D Radon Transform

Bone responses in B-mode US images typically appear as elongated line-like objects with higher intensity values compared to the other image features. Integrating the intensity values along these bone responses in an image will produce a higher value than doing the integration along a non-bone response (Fig. 1). Based on this simple idea, we propose to use the 3D Radon Transform (*3DRT*) in order to detect the orientation and location of the bone surfaces. *3DRT* represents a 3D volume as a collection of projections in a function domain *f(x,y,z)* along various planes defined by the shortest distance ρ from origin, the angle azimuth ϕ around *z* axis and the angle of elevation θ around the *y* axis:

$$3DRT(\rho,\phi,\theta) = \int \int \int f(x,y,z)\delta(\rho - x\cos\phi\cos\theta - y\sin\phi\sin\theta - z\sin\theta)dxdydz. \tag{3}$$

The *3DRT* is calculated for the local phase bone surface points extracted in 2.1. From this point on the *3DRT* volumes will be denoted as $3DRT_{CT}(\rho_{CT},\phi_{CT},\theta_{CT})$ and $3DRT_{US}(\rho_{US},\phi_{US},\theta_{US})$ for the CT and US bone surfaces, respectively.

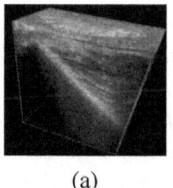 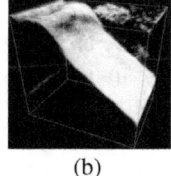 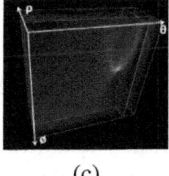

(a)   (b)   (c)

Fig. 1. 3D Radon Transform (3DRT) and bone orientation estimation. (a) B-mode US volume; (b) 3D phase symmetry volume of (a); (c) 3DRT of (b) where the high intensity region is showing a peak (high intensity) in the 3DRT space due to integration of the bone surface for the angle values that are corresponding to the bone surface orientation.

2.3   Projection Based Phase Correlation for CT-US Registration

The *3DRT*s calculated in Section 2.2 are used as the input volumes to the phase correlation based registration method. The rigid body registration problem is solved in two steps: first estimating the 3D rotation, then the 3D translation. In order to calculate the angle difference in the azimuth direction (*z* axis) between the *3DRT_CT* and *3DRT_US* volumes, intensity values along the elevation direction (*y* axis) are summed resulting in two-dimensional (2D) RT images denoted as *2DRT_CTy* (ρ_{CT},ϕ_{CT}) and *2DRT_USy* (ρ_{US},ϕ_{US}), respectively. From properties of RT the relationship between these two RT images is given by:

$$2DRT_{CTy}(\rho_{CT},\phi_{CT}) = 2DRT_{USy}((\rho_{CT} - \Delta\rho_{\phi},\phi_{CT} - \phi). \tag{4}$$

Here, $\Delta\rho_{\phi}=(\Delta x^2 + \Delta y^2)^{0.5}\times sin(\phi\text{-}tan^{-1}(\Delta x /\Delta y))$ where $(\Delta x ,\Delta y)$ is the translational difference in *x* and *y* directions. Let $F_{CTy}(f,\phi_{CT})$ and $F_{USy}(f,\phi_{US})$ denote the one-dimensional (1D) Fourier transforms with respect to the first argument of *2DRT_CTy* and *2DRT_USy*, respectively. For each ϕ_{CT},ϕ_{US} angle combination a projection based phase correlation function is calculated.

$$PC_{rot}(\phi_{CT},\phi_{US}) = \frac{F_{CTy}(f,\phi_{CT}) \times F_{USy}^*(f,\phi_{US})}{\left|F_{CTy}(f,\phi_{CT}) \times F_{USy}^*(f,\phi_{US})\right|}. \tag{5}$$

In Equation (5), F^* denotes the complex conjugate. Next step involves the calculation of the $Peak(\phi_{CT},\phi_{US})=max(IF^{-1}(PC_{rot}(\phi_{CT}, \phi_{US})))$ matrix where IF^{-1} denotes the 1D inverse Fourier transform operation. The $Peak(\phi_{CT}, \phi_{US})$ matrix will have high intensity pixels when $\phi_{CT}=\phi+\phi_{US}$ since the correlation between the *2DRT_CTy* and *2DRT_USy* images will be high for these angles. Thus, we introduce a sum function $Sum_y(a)$:

$$Sum_y(a) = \sum_{\phi} Peak(\phi_{CT},\phi_{CT} - a) \; where \; \phi_{CT} - a \geq 0$$

$$Sum_y(a) = \sum_{\phi} Peak(\phi_{CT}, 180 + \phi_{CT} - a) \; where \; \phi_{CT} - a \leq 0 \tag{6}$$

Function $Sum_y(a)$ will reach a maximum value at $a=\phi$ [14]. Consequently, the rotation angle ϕ is detected by determining the maximum value of $Sum_y(a)$ [14]. After finding the ϕ angle same analysis is repeated to find the rotation difference θ in the elevation direction (*y* axis), this intensity summation is performed along the z axis resulting in 2D *RT* images denoted as *2DRT_CTz* (ρ_{CT},ϕ_{CT}) and *2DRT_USz* (ρ_{US},ϕ_{US}), respectively. The only difference is that this time the intensity summation is performed along the azimuth direction.

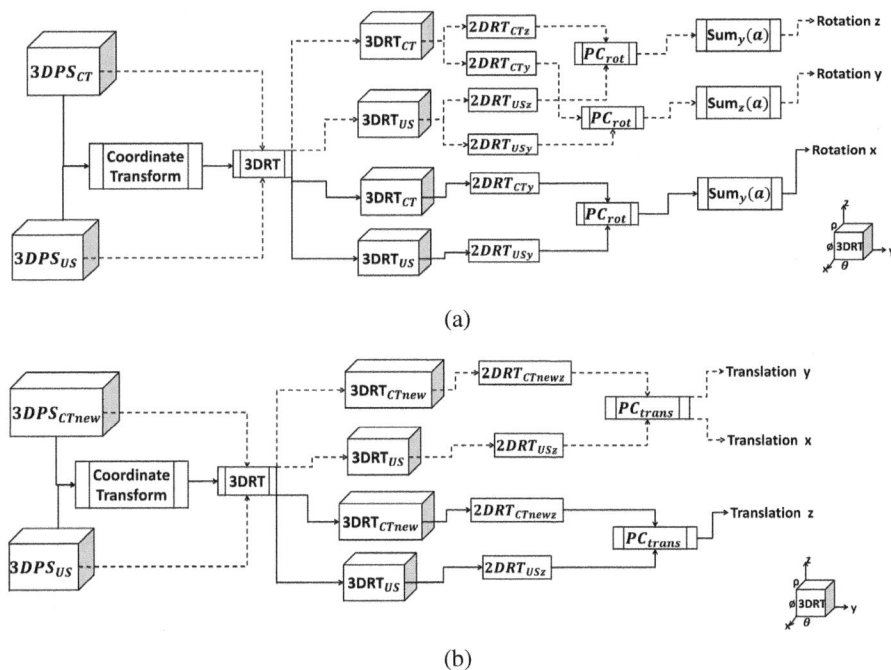

(a)

(b)

Fig. 2. Flowchart for the proposed 3D rotation (a) and translation (b) estimation

The integration in the *3DRT* given in Equation (3) is done along the *y* and *z* axis. In order to calculate the final rotation (rotation around the *x* axis), this integration has to be done around *x* axis. To achieve this a coordinate transformation is done in the original *3DRT$_{US}$* and *3DRT$_{CT}$* volumes making the *x* axis to be represented as the *z* axis in both volumes. Rotation *x* can now be calculated as explained previously for the elevation angle (ø) calculation. The 3D rotation estimation process is shown in Fig.2 (a) as a flowchart.

The calculated angle values are used to correct for the rotational difference between the PS_{3DCT} and PS_{3DUS} volumes. After this correction the only difference between the two local phase volumes is the 3D translational difference. A new *3DRT* is calculated for the rotation corrected local phase volume. Let us symbolize this new *3DRT* volume as *3DRT$_{CTnew}$*. As in the rotation estimation part the new *3DRT$_{CTnew}$* volume is reduced to 2D by summing the intensity values along the azimuth direction (*z* axis). This new 2D image $2DRT_{CTnezz}(\rho_{CT}, \theta)$ and the previously calculated $2DRT_{USz}(\rho_{US}, \theta)$ are used as inputs to the PC_{trans} formula given in Equation (7) below. The angle values in $2DRT_{USz}$ and $2DRT_{CTnewz}$ are the same stating that there is no rotational difference between these two images.

$$PC_{trans}(f, \o) = \frac{F_{USz}(f, \theta) \times F^*_{CTnewz}(f, \theta)}{|F_{USz}(f, \theta) \times F^*_{CTnewz}(f, \theta)|}. \qquad (7)$$

Again, $F_{USz}(f,\theta)$ and $F_{CTnewz}(f,\theta)$ denote the one dimensional (1D) Fourier transforms of $2DRT_{USz}$ and $2DRT_{CTnewz}$, respectively, whereas F^* denotes the complex conjugate. Next step involves the calculation 1D inverse Fourier transform of $PC_{trans}(f,\theta)$ in order to obtain $pc_{trans}(\rho,\theta)= IF^{-1}(PC_{trans}(f,\theta))$.

From Equation (4), we know that this function will have high intensity values when $\rho_{CT}=(\Delta x^2+ \Delta y^2)^{0.5}\times sin(\phi\text{-}tan^{-1}(\Delta x /\Delta y))$ since the correlation between the reference and floating images will be the highest for these ρ_{CT} values. In order to find the translational displacement in x and y directions the final step involves taking the inverse RT of $pc_{trans}(\rho,\theta)$ and searching the maximum peak value of $H(x,y)=2DRT^{-1}$ $(pc_{trans}(\rho,\theta))$. Here, $2DRT^{-1}$ denotes the inverse RT operation. The translation in the z direction is calculated using the same method after the coordinate transformation operation to the $3DRT_{CTnew}$ and $3DRT_{US}$ volumes [14]. Fig. 2 (b) shows a simple flowchart of the 3D translation estimation method.

2.4   Data Acquisition and Experimental Setup

A Sawbones pelvis bone model (#1301, Research Laboratories, Inc., Vashon, WA) was used during the phantom validation experiment. 38 fiducial markers with 1 mm diameter were attached to the surface of the phantom specifically covering the iliac and pubic crest regions. This phantom setup was immersed inside a water tank and imaged with a GE Voluson 730 Expert Ultrasound Machine (GE Healthcare, Waukesha, WI) using a 3D RSP4-12 probe. The US phantom volumes were 152×198×148 voxels with an isometric resolution of 0.24 mm. The CT volume was taken with a Toshiba Aquilion 64 (Tustin, CA). The voxel resolution was 0.76 mm×0.76 mm×0.3 mm. The 3DRT was implemented in C++. Local phase bone surface extraction together with the registration method was implemented in Matlab (The Mathworks Inc., Natick, MA, USA). The US and CT volumes were initially aligned using the gold standard for registration calculated from fiducial markers. The CT volume was then perturbed by a random transform chosen from a uniform distribution of ±10 mm translation along each axis and ±10° rotation about each axis. In total 100 different distributions were introduced to the CT volume. The misaligned CT volumes were then registered back to the US volume using our proposed registration algorithm. Accuracy was determined by the ability of the registration to recover to the fiducial-based gold standard and is reported as the mean Target Registration Error (TRE) calculated as the misalignment of the four new fiducals, which were not included in the initial fiducial based registration. The Surface Registration Error (SRE) was calculated as the Root Mean Square (rms) distance between the registered surfaces.

Following all required ethics approvals, we also obtained both CT and US scans from consenting patients admitted to a Level 1 Trauma Centre with pelvic fractures that clinically require a CT scan. The voxel resolution for the CT volumes varied between 0.76 mm-0.83 mm in x and y axes and 1 mm-2 mm in z. The US volumes were acquired using the same US machine as described in the phantom study. In total six patients were scanned. The RMS error between the registered bone surface volumes was used for quantitative validation.

3   Results

Figure 3 shows the registration results for one of the introduced misalignments in the phantom study. During the registration process the entire left pelvis was used as the CT surface and no ROI was defined. The proposed registration method successfully aligns the two volumes where a close match between the surfaces is visible (Fig.3.). The tests on the phantom setup showed an average 2.06 mm (SD 0.59 mm) TRE with maximum TRE of 3.34 mm. The mean surface registration error for the phantom study was calculated as 0.8 mm (SD 0.62 mm).

Figure 4 shows the qualitative results obtained from the clinical study. The US scans were obtained from the healthy (unaffected by the fracture) side of the pelvis. The mean SRE, obtained from the six patients, was 0.74 (SD 0.22 mm) with maximum SRE of 1.1 mm. The runtime for the 3D RT for a 400×400×400 volume is 4 min. The MATLAB implementation of the registration method takes 2 min.

4   Discussion and Conclusion

We proposed a method for CT-US registration that is based on aligning local phase based bone features in frequency domain using their projections. Unlike the previous approaches the proposed method is fully automatic, non-iterative and requires no initial alignment between the two datasets. Using local phase images as input images to PC method eliminates the typical edge effect problem, which is one of the main problems faced in PC based registration methods. The use of RT in order to estimate the rotation proved to be very robust specifically in bone US images. During the traditional Fourier Transform based registration algorithms the rotation is estimated by transforming Cartesian coordinates to polar coordinates. During this transformation image pixels close to the center are oversampled while image pixels further away from the center are under sampled or missed, which causes problems for rotation estimation. On the other hand, RT concentrates on the image regions where high feature information is available, which makes the method more robust to rotation estimation.

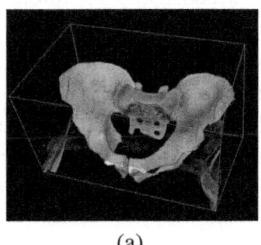 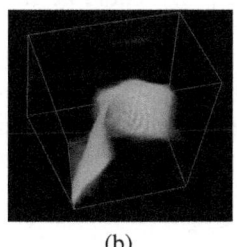 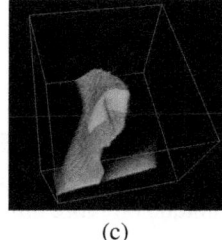

(a)   (b)   (c)

Fig. 3. Qualitative validation for phantom study. (a) 3D phase symmetry surface of phantom pelvis; (b) 3D local phase symmetry surface; (c) shows the obtained registration result where (a) is registered to (b). Note that the entire left pelvis is used for registration and no ROI was selected.

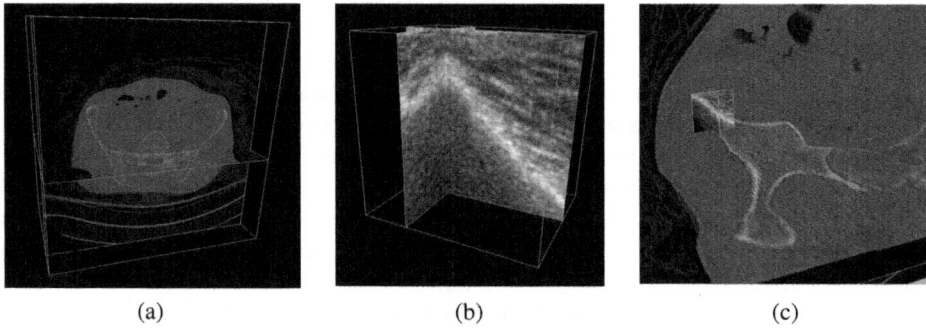

Fig. 4. Qualitative validation for clinical study. (a) CT data obtained from a pelvic ring fracture patient; (b) corresponding 3D US volume; (c) overlay of registration result.

The calculation of RT requires some discretization as well which could potentially introduce some errors. Recently, sparsity based image processing techniques have shown to improve the calculation of the RT [15]. This will be further investigated as a future step. Furthermore, in US based orthopaedic surgery applications the bone surfaces typically appear as elongated line-like features. This information was incorporated into the proposed framework using the traditional RT where the intensity integration was performed along a line. In order to enhance bone features or soft tissue interfaces that have a curved appearance this traditional RT could be extended to generalized RT where the integration would be performed alone a curve.

One limitation of the proposed method is its dependency on the extracted local phase features. Since US is a user dependent imaging modality the proper orientation of the US transducer plays an important role during the data collection. If the transducer is aligned properly, the bone surface will be represented with a high intensity line-like region followed by a shadowing feature which results in the accurate extraction of local phase bone surfaces. On the other hand, wrong orientation of the transducer will result in weak bone responses which will also affect the extracted local phase bone features. In these situations the proposed method could be used as an initial registration step that could be further optimized using an intensity based method followed by this initial registration.

We believe that the registration time could be reduced by implementing the method on a Graphics Processing Unit (GPU). While the registration procedure has shown promise in the tests, it still requires further improvements to the implementation and must be further validated to be ready for a clinical application. Future work will focus on reducing the registration runtime and on extensive validation of the registration technique on more clinical scans.

Acknowledgments. This work was funded by Mprime Network.

References

1. Nolte, L.P., Zamorano, L.J., Jiang, Z., Wang, Q., Langlotz, F., Berlemann, F.: Image-guided insertion of transpedicular screws. A Laboratory Set-Up. Spine 20(4), 497–500 (1995)
2. Jaramaz, B., DiGioia, A.M., Blackwell, M., Nikou, C.: Computer assisted measurement of cup placement in total hip replacement. Clinical Orthopaedics 354, 70–81 (1998)
3. Tyryshkin, K., Mousavi, P., Beek, M., Ellis, R., Dichora, P., Abolmaesumi, P.: A navigation system for shoulder arthroscopic surgery. Journal of Engineering in Medicine: Special Issue on Navigation Systems in Computer-assisted Orthopaedic Surgery, 801–812 (2007)
4. Hacihaliloglu, I., Abugharbieh, R., Hodgson, A., Rohling, R.: Bone Surface Localization in Ultrasound Using Image Phase Based Features. Ultrasound in Med. and Biol. 35(9), 1475–1487 (2009)
5. Penney, G.P., Edwards, P.J., King, A.P., Blackall, J.M., Batchelor, P.G., Hawkes, D.J.: A Stochastic Iterative Closest Point Algorithm (stochastICP). In: Niessen, W.J., Viergever, M.A. (eds.) MICCAI 2001. LNCS, vol. 2208, pp. 762–769. Springer, Heidelberg (2001)
6. Moghari, M.H., Abolmaesumi, P.: Point-Based Rigid-Body Registration Using an Unscented Kalman Filter. IEEE Transactions on Medical Imaging 26(12), 1708–1728 (2007)
7. Brounstein, A., Hacihaliloglu, I., Guy, P., Hodgson, A., Abugharbieh, R.: Towards Real-Time 3D US to CT Bone Image Registration Using Phase and Curvature Feature Based GMM Matching. In: Fichtinger, G., Martel, A., Peters, T. (eds.) MICCAI 2011, Part I. LNCS, vol. 6891, pp. 235–242. Springer, Heidelberg (2011)
8. Brendel, B., Winter, S., Rick, A., Stockheim, M., Ermert, H.: Registration of 3D CT and Ultrasound Datasets of the Spine Using Bone Structures. Computer Aided Surgery 7, 146–155 (2002)
9. Penney, G., Barratt, D., Chan, C., Slomczykowski, M., Carter, T., Edwards, P., Hawkes, D.: Cadaver Validation of Intensity-Based Ultrasound to CT Registration. Medical Image Analysis 10(3), 385–395 (2006)
10. Gill, S., Abolmaesumi, P., Fichtinger, G., Boisvert, J., Pichora, D., Borshneck, D., Mousavi, P.: Biomechanically Constrained Groupwise Ultrasound to CT Registration of the Lumbar Spine. Medical Image Analysis (2010) (in Press)
11. Khallaghi, S., Mousavi, P., Borschneck, D., Fichtinger, G., Abolmaesumi, P.: Biomechanically Constrained Groupwise Statistical Shape Model to Ultrasound Registration of the Lumbar Spine. In: Taylor, R.H., Yang, G.-Z. (eds.) IPCAI 2011. LNCS, vol. 6689, pp. 47–54. Springer, Heidelberg (2011)
12. Foroughi, P., Boctor, E., Swatrz, M.J., Taylor, R.H., Fichtinger, G.: Ultrasound bone segmentation using dynamic programming. In: IEEE Ultrasonics Syposium, pp. 2523–2526 (2007)
13. Hacihaliloglu, I., Abugharbieh, R., Hodgson, A.J., Rohling, R.: Automatic Bone Localization and Fracture Detection from Volumetric Ultrasound Images Using 3D Local Phase Features. Ultrasound in Medicine and Biology 38(1), 128–144 (2011)
14. Tsuboi, T., Hirai, S.: Detection of Planar Motion Objects Using Radon Transform and One-Dimensional Phase-Only Matched Filtering. Systems and Computers in Japan 37(5), 1963–1972 (2006)
15. Gurbuz, A.C., McClellan, J.H., Romberg, J., Scott, W.R.: Compressive sensing of parameterized shapes in images. In: Proceedings of IEEE International Conference on Acoustics, Speech and Signal Processing, pp. 1949–1952 (2008)

A Hierarchical Strategy for Reconstruction of 3D Acetabular Surface Models from 2D Calibrated X-Ray Images

Steffen Schumann[1], Moritz Tannast[2], Mathias Bergmann[3], Michael Thali[4],
Lutz-P. Nolte[1], and Guoyan Zheng[1]

[1] Institute for Surgical Technology and Biomechanics, University of Bern,
Switzerland
[2] Inselspital, Orthopaedic Department, University of Bern, Switzerland
[3] Institute of Anatomy, University of Bern, Switzerland
[4] Institute of Forensic Medicine, University of Bern, Switzerland

Abstract. Recent studies have shown the advantage of performing range of motion experiments based on three-dimensional (3D) bone models to diagnose femoro-acetabular impingement (FAI). The relative motion of pelvic and femoral surface models is assessed dynamically in order to analyze potential bony conflicts. 3D surface models are normally retrieved by 3D imaging modalities like computed tomography (CT) or magnetic resonance imaging (MRI). Despite the obvious advantage of using these modalities, surgeons still rely on the acquisition of planar X-ray radiographs to diagnose orthopedic impairments like FAI. Although X-ray imaging has advantages such as accessibility, inexpensiveness and low radiation exposure, it only provides two-dimensional information. Therefore, a 3D reconstruction of the hip joint based on planar X-ray radiographs would bring an enormous benefit for diagnosis and planning of FAI-related problems. In this paper we present a new approach to calibrate conventional X-ray images and to reconstruct a 3D surface model of the acetabulum. Starting from the registration of a statistical shape model (SSM) of the hemi-pelvis, a localized patch-SSM is matched to the calibrated X-ray scene in order to recover the acetabular shape. We validated the proposed approach with X-ray radiographs acquired from 6 different cadaveric hips.

1 Introduction

Three-dimensionally (3D) reconstructed bone shapes are an important means for clinical diagnosis of orthopedic impairments [1][2]. 3D bone shapes are normally retrieved from computed-tomography (CT) datasets by performing semi-automatic segmentation. However, in order to reduce costs and to keep the radiation exposure to the patient low, the acquisition of planar X-ray radiographs is in general preferred to CT-scans. Based on the 2D X-ray projections of the anatomy, important clinical parameters are estimated to make a diagnosis or to plan a surgical treatment.

P. Abolmaesumi et al. (Eds.): IPCAI 2012, LNAI 7330, pp. 74–83, 2012.

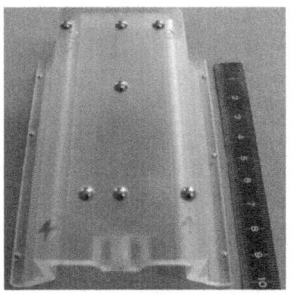 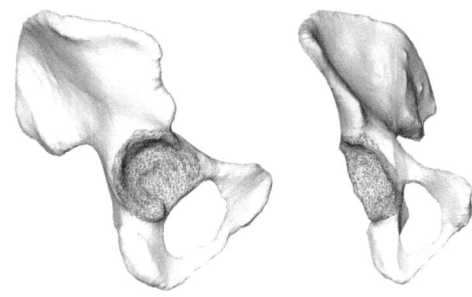

Fig. 1. Left: Topview of calibration phantom showing top layer with seven fiducials. Right: Definition of acetabulum patch based on mean hemi-pelvis model.

X-ray images also play a major role in the diagnosis of femoro-acetabular impingement (FAI). In order to identify possible bony conflicts between acetabular structures of the pelvis and the proximal femur, an anterior-posterior (AP) and a cross-table axial X-ray radiograph are normally acquired [3]. Special attention has to be paid to the correct alignment of the patient's hip joint with respect to the image plane. Otherwise, wrong interpretations or miscalculations could occur [4]. Moreover, X-ray projections only provide two-dimensional (2D) information. Recent trials have shown an improvement in FAI diagnosis and planning by performing range of motion studies using 3D surface models of the pelvis and the proximal femur, which are normally derived from 3D imaging modalities such as CT or MRI [4,5]. However, in clinical routine, CT-scans are only acquired in rare cases of severe pelvic deformations [6] and magnetic-resonance imaging (MRI) poses a challenge for 3D bone segmentation. In this paper, we propose to derive 3D information from two X-ray images.

In previous work we have already successfully shown that it is possible to reconstruct the 3D surface of the proximal femur from calibrated X-ray images with a sufficient accuracy [7]. In the following, we are going to describe a method to reconstruct the 3D shape of the acetabulum from biplanar radiographs. The major challenge is thereby to recover the correct fossa depth and the rim curvatures. Besides the development of a small-sized mobile X-ray calibration phantom, a hierarchical strategy was developed to precisely reconstruct the shape of the acetabulum. Our approach was validated based on six pairs of X-ray radiographs, acquired from six dry cadaveric bones.

2 Materials and Methods

2.1 Calibration

A calibration step is required in order to extract quantitative information from 2D X-ray projections. This step is accomplished by integrating a mobile phantom (Fig. 1) into the X-ray imaging process. The phantom is designed to have 16 fiducials of two different dimensions embedded, arranged in three different planes.

The 3D locations of these fiducials are determined in the coordinate-system of the reference-base attached to the calibration phantom using a tracked pointer. The 2D image locations of the fiducials are determined based on the inherent geometric arrangement of the fiducial spheres and image processing steps. Based on simple thresholding and connected-component labeling methods, candidate fiducials are extracted from the image. In order to identify correct fiducial detections and to establish correspondences between all the 2D and 3D fiducial locations, a lookup-table (LUT) based strategy has been developed. A prerequisite for this strategy is the successful detection of one of the line patterns in the top layer of the phantom (Fig. 1). The detected line pattern is then used to normalize all the detected candidate fiducials. These normalized positions are then compared with an off-line generated LUT consisting of simulated fiducial projections with different extrinsic calibration parameters. In order to identify the optimal LUT item, a distance map is computed between all the LUT items and the current set of normalized fiducial positions. Cross-correlation is further applied to identify the precise fiducial positions derived from the optimal LUT-item. The calibration parameters are then computed based on commonly used direct linear transformation method [8]. For detailed information on the phantom detection algorithm we would like to refer to our work [9].

2.2   Patch Statistical Shape Model Construction

Statistical shape models (SSMs) have been originally introduced by Cootes et al. [10] to the field of image processing. Based on a training population of shape instances, its statistical variation can be used to derive new valid shapes. A SSM of the hemi-pelvis (one for each patient side) was constructed from a training population $m = 20$ CT-datasets. Surface model instances were semi-automatically segmented and extracted using Amira software (Visage Imaging, Richmond, Australia). Direct correspondences between the instances were established using diffeomorphic demons algorithm [11]. The intensity-based method was used to register the binary segmentation volumes of the corresponding pelvis surface models, whereas each aligned surface instance $X^{I,r}$ consists of N 3D vertices:

$$X^{I,r} = \{X_0^{I,r}, Y_0^{I,r}, Z_0^{I,r}, \ldots, X_n^{I,r}, Y_n^{I,r}, Z_n^{I,r}, \ldots, X_{N-1}^{I,r}, Y_{N-1}^{I,r}, Z_{N-1}^{I,r}\} \quad (1)$$

where I denotes the specific instance and $r \in \{\text{left}, \text{right}\}$ represents the pelvis side. Principal component analysis (PCA) was then applied to the aligned training population to explore the statistical variability (Fig. 2). For a proper clinical diagnosis of FAI related problems, the main interest is in the 3D shape of the hip joint. Hence, the focus here is on the 3D reconstruction of the acetabular shape. In order to accomplish this, an acetabular patch-SSM was constructed for each patient side. The patch-SSM concept has been originally introduced in [12][13] in order to guide the matching of a pelvis-SSM to sparse ultrasound data. In the present study, we will apply it for reconstruction of 3D acetabular surface models from 2D calibrated X-ray images.

Based on the mean hemi-pelvis model $\overline{X}^r$ of the training population, the acetabulum patch was interactively defined. Thereby, mainly the fossa region

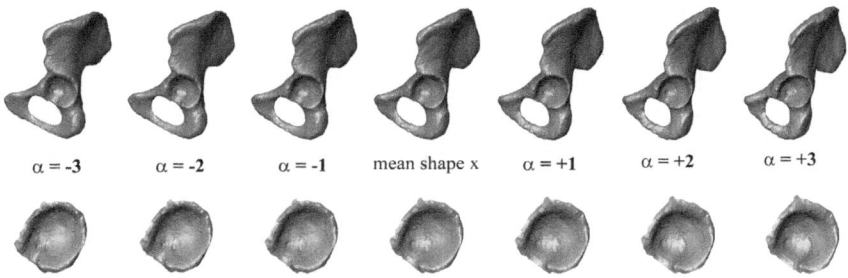

Fig. 2. First eigenmode of variations of the left hemi-pelvis (first row) and of the left acetabulum-patch (second row), generated by evaluating $y + \alpha\sqrt{\lambda_j}p_j$ with $\alpha \in \{-3, \ldots, +3\}$, $y = \{\overline{X}, \overline{q}\}$, eigenvectors p_j and eigenvalues λ_j

and the acetabular rim were selected as shown in Fig. 1, resulting in a list of K numbered vertices:

$$v^r = \{v_0^r, v_1^r, \ldots, v_k^r, \ldots, v_{K-1}^r\} \tag{2}$$

where $v_k = \{n\}$. As correspondences between all training instances were established in a previous step (Eq. 1), an acetabulum surface patch $q^{I,r}$ could be extracted from the associated hemi-pelvis model $X^{I,r}$ using the list of numbered vertices:

$$q^{I,r} = \{q_0^{I,r}, q_1^{I,r}, \ldots, q_k^{I,r}, \ldots, q_{K-1}^{I,r}\} \tag{3}$$

where $q_k^{I,r} = \{X_{v_k^r}^{I,r}, Y_{v_k^r}^{I,r}, Z_{v_k^r}^{I,r}\}$. In order to compensate for the inherent translational differences of the patch instances $q^{I,r}$, another registration step was performed. This step is required for capturing the local shape variations of the acetabulum. Therefore, the mean patch model $\overline{q}^r$ was extracted from the mean hemi-pelvis model $\overline{X}^r$ according to Eq. 3:

$$\overline{q}^r = \{\overline{q}_0^r, \overline{q}_1^r, \ldots, \overline{q}_k^r, \ldots, \overline{q}_{K-1}^r\} \tag{4}$$

where $\overline{q}_k^r = \{\overline{X}_{v_k^r}^r, \overline{Y}_{v_k^r}^r, \overline{Z}_{v_k^r}^r\}$. In the following, each patch instance $q^{I,r}$ was rigidly registered to the mean patch $\overline{q}^r$. Afterwards, PCA was applied again to reveal the statistical variability. The first eigenmode of the acetabulum patch-SSM is depicted in Fig. 2.

2.3   3D Acetabular Shape Reconstruction

In the following description, we denote the bone edges extracted from the 2D X-ray images as contours and the corresponding apparent contours extracted from a 3D model (mean surface model or an instantiated model) as silhouettes.

Feature Extraction. In order to register a SSM to the X-ray radiographs, certain pelvic features have to be extracted from both images. After calibrating both images, the anterior superior iliac spine (ASIS), the pubis symphysis and the posterior inferior iliac spine (PIIS) landmarks of the respective hemi-pelvis have to be defined on both radiographs. As these landmarks are normally difficult to identify in the axial image, the landmarks are first determined in the AP image. As a calibration is available, we could find the epipolar lines of these landmarks on the axial radiograph [8]. These epipolar lines can be used to guide the identification of the corresponding landmarks in the axial image (top-left image in Fig. 3).

Moreover, certain pelvic contours need to be defined semi-automatically. This step is performed using live-wire algorithm as implemented in VTK-library[1]. The following four image contours of the respective hemi-pelvis need to be determined (top row images of Fig. 3):

o contour of hemi-pelvis
o anterior contour of the acetabular rim
o posterior contour of the acetabular rim
o contour of acetabular fossa

Hierarchical Patch-SSM Based Registration. After the semi-automatic extraction of the pelvic features, the remaining steps of statistical shape model registration are automatically performed. In the first place, the mean hemi-pelvis model $\overline{X}^r$ is registered to the X-ray scene using paired-point matching. The corresponding landmarks (see previous section 2.3) were predefined based on the mean hemi-pelvis model and used to compute the affine transformation from the hemi-pelvis SSM space to the X-ray space. The alignment of the hemi-pelvis SSM was further improved based on the 3-stage approach by Zheng et al. [14]. This approach is based on finding correspondences between the silhouettes of the surface model (here: the silhouettes of the mean hemi-pelvis model $\overline{X}^r$) and the 2D outer contours of the projected surface model (here: the contours of the hemi-pelvis defined in both X-ray images). These correspondences are then used to estimate the affine transformation between the two spaces. This registration step is followed by a statistical instantiation and regularized non-rigid deformation. After completion of the 3-stage based alignment, an optimal match of the hemi-pelvis SSM to the X-ray scene is achieved. However, the match is only based on the outer contour of the pelvis, as extracted from the X-ray images.

In order to improve the fitting around the acetabular region, information on additional contours of the acetabulum needs to be integrated. Besides the anterior and posterior acetabular rim contours also the fossa contour can be identified. As the fossa of the hemi-pelvis does not provide a visible silhouette, matching cannot be established. Therefore, the instantiated hemi-pelvis model is replaced by the mean surface model of the acetabular patch-SSM based on the direct correspondences according to Eq. 3. This localized patch-SSM is more suitable to be registered to the additional X-ray contours of the acetabulum, as all the relevant silhouettes can be easily extracted.

After aligning the patch-SSM with respect to the X-ray scene based on the in-stantiated hemi-pelvis model, a scaled rigid transformation based on the

---

[1] Visualization Toolkit; www.vtk.org

anterior and posterior acetabular rim contours and their corresponding silhouettes is further estimated. These silhouettes were defined a priori based on the
mean patch model and were used to establish correspondences with the respective contours defined in X-ray images. It was found that an initial scale estimation is critical for an accurate reconstruction of the acetabular surface model.
In the present study, this was done as follows. All the anterior and posterior
acetabular rim contours (silhouettes) in X-ray (SSM-) space were treated as one
point set, whereas the unit of the contour points is in *pixels* and the unit of the
silhouette points is in *mm*. For each of the three point sets (there were 2D contour point sets, one from the AP image and the other from the axial image, and
one 3D silhouette point set from the mean patch model), the first principal axis
was computed. Subsequently, the points were projected on this principal axis
and the distances $d_c^{AP,axial}$ ($d_s^{AP,axial}$) between two contour (silhouette) points
farthest away along the axis were determined. The average distance d_c for both
images was further multiplied by the pixel scaling factor, determined from the
calibration procedure, to convert it from *pixel* to *mm* unit. The initial scale was
then determined as the ratio between d_c and d_s.

In order to recover the acetabular depth, the registration is further extended
by involving the fossa region. Correspondences of the fossa region in X-ray and
SSM-space are determined iteratively. For each step, all points of the fossa contour in X-ray space are backprojected using the calibration matrix, resulting
in 3D rays. For each ray, the distances to all mean patch model vertices are
computed. The vertex with minimal Euclidean distance to the 3D ray is taken
as corresponding point to the respective fossa contour point in X-ray space.
Together with the corresponding point pairs of the anterior and posterior acetabular rim points, an affine registration is computed to update the position
and scale of the mean patch model with respect to all three contours. The 3D
reconstruction of the acetabulum is completed by statistical instantiation [15] of
the patch-SSM taking all three contours into consideration.

2.4   Experiments and Results

The proposed hierarchical strategy for acetabulum reconstruction was tested on
six cadaveric bones (none of the bones was involved in the SSM construction
process). Six pairs of X-ray radiographs (anterior-posterior and cross-table axial) were acquired, whereas both hip joints were considered for reconstruction of
the acetabulum. Prior to the X-ray acquisition, the calibration phantom, the femur bone and the pelvis were equipped with passive reference bases and tracked
during acquisition by an infrared camera system (Polaris, NDI, Canada), as the
bones and the phantom were subject to movement during the image acquisition.
The acquired images were calibrated individually with respect to the coordinate system established by the reference base attached to the pelvis and the
features were semi-automatically determined according to section 2.3. While the
determination of the landmarks and acetabular contours took about 1 minute
per image, the extraction of hemi-pelvis contours took about 2-3 minutes per
image.The 3D reconstruction of the acetabular surface was then performed au-

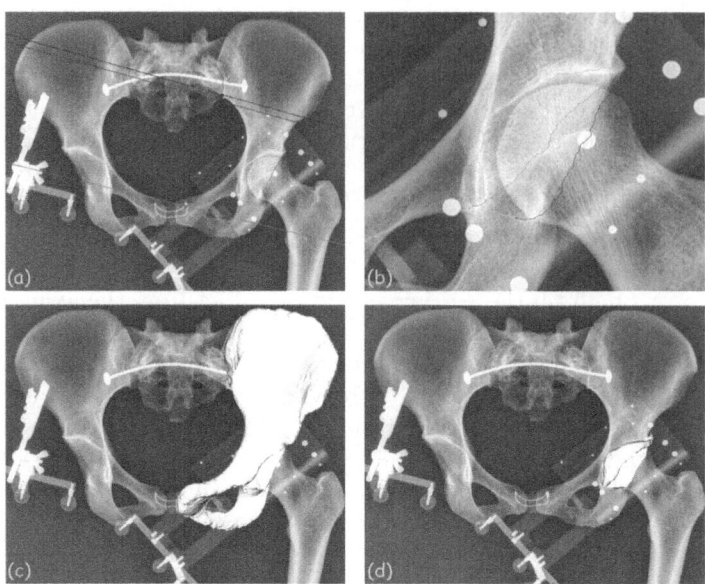

Fig. 3. Hierarchical 2D/3D reconstruction strategy: (a) contour of hemi-pelvis and landmarks with epipolar lines (green: pubis symphysis, red: ASIS, blue: PIIS) (b) acetabular contours (red: posterior rim contour, green: anterior rim contour, cyan: acetabular fossa contour) (c) registered hemi-pelvis SSM (d) registered acetabular patch-SSM

tomatically as described in section 2.3. In order to determine the reconstruction accuracy, CT-scans of the cadaveric pelvises were acquired. The pelvic surface models were extracted from the associated CT-scans and the correspondences between these surface models and the associated mean hemi-pelvis model were established using diffeomorphic demons algorithm [11]. Analogously, acetabulum patches were extracted for both sides and further served as ground truth for validation. On the basis of the direct correspondences, the ground truth acetabulum was rigidly registered to the corresponding reconstructed 3D acetabular surface. The reconstruction accuracy was then assessed using MESH-tool [16], which uses the Hausdorff distance to estimate the distance between triangular 3D meshes. Two experiments were performed to evaluate the efficacy of the present approach.

In the first experiment, the accuracy of deriving the acetabular surface models only based on the hemi-pelvis reconstruction was evaluated. For each case, an acetabulum patch was directly extracted from the reconstructed hemi-pelvis model based on direct correspondences (Eq. 3). In the second experiment, we analyzed the accuracy of the present method. For each experiment, twelve reconstructed acetabular surface models were obtained and compared to the associated ground truth surface models. An overview of the complete error distribution of the twelve reconstructed acetabular surface models in each experiment is presented with box plot. The box plot in Fig. 4 represents the error distribution

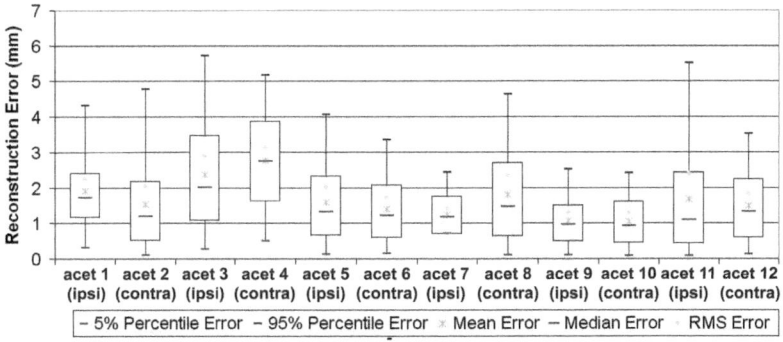

Fig. 4. Box plot indicating the accuracy of the twelve acetabular surface models extracted from the reconstructed hemi-pelvis models

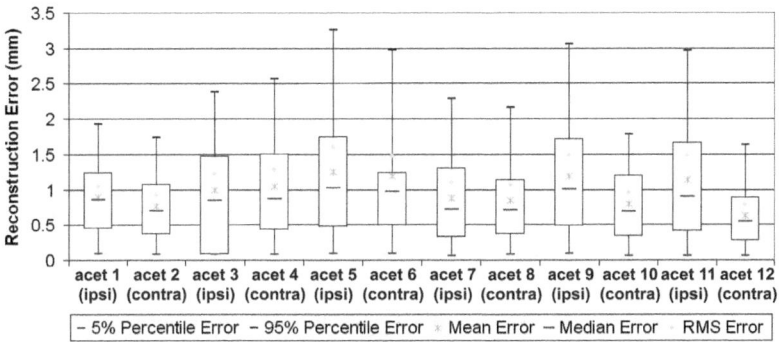

Fig. 5. Box plot indicating the accuracy of the present method

of the first experiment, while Fig. 5 shows the error distribution of the second experiment. For all datasets the mean error, root mean squared (RMS) error as well as the 5%, 25%, 50%, 75% and 95% percentile errors were computed. The average mean error of the 12 acetabular surface models obtained from the reconstructed hemi-pelvis models was 1.659 ± 0.508 mm and this error decreased to 0.970 ± 0.198 mm when the present method was used. On average, the present method improved the reconstruction accuracy by 0.688 mm. It was found that the present method unanimously improved the acetabular surface model reconstruction accuracy for almost all datasets except one dataset (*acet9*), where the accuracy was slightly worse. Regions of error occurred either in the fossa (dataset *acet2* in Fig. 6), or at the cutting edge of the patch (dataset *acet12* in Fig. 6), but rarely along the acetabular rim (dataset *acet1* in Fig. 6).

The X-ray image acquisition was always focused on one pelvis side. The calibration phantom was arranged with respect to the hip joint of the focused side (e.g. left patient side in Fig. 3). In order to investigate an impact of calibration phantom positioning on the reconstruction accuracy, the reconstruction errors

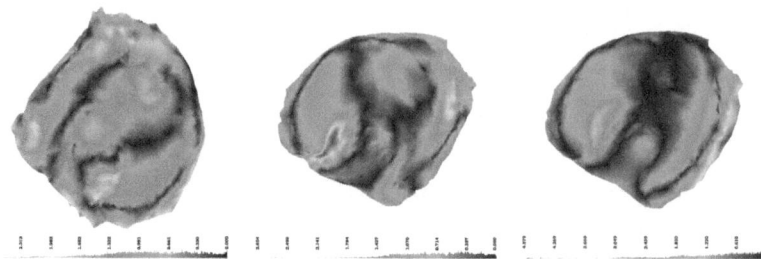

Fig. 6. Analysis of reconstruction accuracy using MESH-tool [16]. The error values are superimposed on the reconstructed acetabular surface models. Datasets, depicted from left to right: acet1, acet2 & acet11.

of ipsi- (when phantom was positioned close to the acetabulum to be reconstructed) and contralateral (when phantom was positioned on contralateral side of the pelvis) side were compared. While the mean reconstruction error for the ipsilateral cases is 1.061 ± 0.159 mm, the mean error for the contralateral cases is 0.879 ± 0.203 mm. For the acquired six datasets, the reconstruction is slightly better for the contralateral side although the exact reason for this needs to be carefully analyzed in the future when more data will be available.

3   Discussion

A 3D reconstruction of the hip joint from conventional X-ray radiographs would have an enormous benefit for the diagnosis and planning of FAI-related issues. Therefore, we proposed a method for X-ray calibration and subsequent acetabular 2D/3D reconstruction. We developed a mobile X-ray calibration phantom, which can be placed anywhere next to the hip joint. It does not interfere the image acquisition and is thus regarded as clinically acceptable. The calibrated images are use to semi-automatically extract relevant pelvic features. The non-rigidly registered hemi-pelvis model is then used to guide the matching of a localized patch-SSM of the acetabulum. Based on the 2D detected acetabular contours, the patch-SSM is optimally fitted to contours extracted from the X-ray images. The proposed method was evaluated based on twelve datasets, acquired from six cadaveric hip joints, showing reasonably good results. Though the clinical significance has not been evaluated, a more accurate reconstruction of the acetabular surface will definitely have a positive impact on the clinical decision.

The main drawbacks of our approach are the user interactivity for contour detection and the required tracking of the patient. However, as a live-wire based semi-automatic method was used to extract the relevant contours, the manual burden on the surgeon is low. Also the presence of soft tissue in clinical cases and possible occlusions of anatomical features by the calibration phantom should not affect the contour extraction, assuming a careful user interaction. The tracking requirement can be omitted by maintaining a fixed relationship between the calibration phantom and the patient.

References

1. Wicky, S., Blaser, P., et al.: Comparison between standard radiography and spiral CT with 3D reconstruction in the evaluation, classification and management of tibial plateau fractures. Eur. Radiol. 10, 1227–1232 (2000)
2. Mitton, D., Zhao, K.: 3D reconstruction of the ribs from lateral and frontal x-rays in comparison to 3D CT-scan reconstruction. J. Biomech. 41, 706–710 (2008)
3. Tannast, M., Siebenrock, K., Anderson, S.: Femoroacetabular impingement: Radiographic diagnosis - what the radiologists should know. AIH Am. J. Roentgenol. 188, 1540–1552 (2007)
4. Krekel, P., Vochteloo, A., et al.: Femoroacetabular impingement and its implications on range of motion: a case report. J. Med. Case Reports 5 (2011)
5. Tannast, M., Goricki, D., et al.: Hip damage occurs at the zone of femoroacetabular impingement. Clin. Orthop. Relat. Res. 466, 273–280 (2008)
6. Beaule, P., Zaragoza, E., et al.: Three-dimensional computed tomography of the hip in the assessment of femoroacetabular impingement. J. Orthop. Res. 23, 1286–1292 (2005)
7. Zheng, G., Schumann, S.: 3D reconstruction of a patient-specific surface model of the proximal femur from calibrated x-ray radiographs: a validation study. Med. Phys. 36, 1155–1166 (2009)
8. Hartley, R., Zisserman, A.: Multiple view geometry in computer vision, 2nd edn. Cambridge University Press (2004)
9. Schumann, S., Dong, X., et al.: Calibration of C-arm for orthopedic interventions via statistical model-based distortion correction and robust phantom detection. In: ISBI. IEEE (2012)
10. Cootes, T., Taylor, C., et al.: Active shape models - their training and application. Comput. Vis. Image Underst. 61, 38–59 (1995)
11. Vercauteren, T., Pennec, X., Perchant, A., Ayache, N.: Non-parametric Diffeomorphic Image Registration with the Demons Algorithm. In: Ayache, N., Ourselin, S., Maeder, A. (eds.) MICCAI 2007, Part II. LNCS, vol. 4792, pp. 319–326. Springer, Heidelberg (2007)
12. Schumann, S., Puls, M., Ecker, T., Schwaegli, T., Stifter, J., Siebenrock, K.-A., Zheng, G.: Determination of Pelvic Orientation from Ultrasound Images Using Patch-SSMs and a Hierarchical Speed of Sound Compensation Strategy. In: Navab, N., Jannin, P. (eds.) IPCAI 2010. LNCS, vol. 6135, pp. 157–167. Springer, Heidelberg (2010)
13. Schumann, S., Nolte, L., Zheng, G.: Compensation of sound speed deviations in 3D B-mode ultrasound for intraoperative determination of the anterior pelvic plane. IEEE Trans. on Inf. Technol. in Biomed. 16, 88–97 (2012)
14. Zheng, G., Rajamani, K.T., Nolte, L.-P.: Use of a Dense Surface Point Distribution Model in a Three-Stage Anatomical Shape Reconstruction from Sparse Information for Computer Assisted Orthopaedic Surgery: A Preliminary Study. In: Narayanan, P.J., Nayar, S.K., Shum, H.-Y. (eds.) ACCV 2006. LNCS, vol. 3852, pp. 52–60. Springer, Heidelberg (2006)
15. Rajamani, K., Styner, M., et al.: Statistical deformable bone models for robust 3D surface extrapolation from sparse data. Med. Image Anal. 11, 99–109 (2007)
16. Aspert, N., Santa-Cruz, D., Ebrahimi, T.: MESH: Measuring errors between surfaces using the Hausdorff distance. In: IEEE International Conference on Multimedia and Expo., vol. 1, pp. 705–708 (2002)

A Navigation Platform for Guidance of Beating Heart Transapical Mitral Valve Repair

John Moore[1], Chris Wedlake[1], Daniel Bainbridge[2], Gerard Guiraudon[2],
Michael Chu[2], Bob Kiaii[2], Pencilla Lang[1], Martin Rajchl[1], and Terry Peters[1]

[1] Western University, Robarts Research Institute, London, Ontario, Canada
{jmoore,cwedlake,tpeters}@robarts.ca, {plang,mrajchl}@imaging.robarts.ca
http://www.robarts.imaging.ca/~tpeters
[2] London Health Sciences Center, London, Ontario, Canada
{Daniel.Bainbridge,Gerard.Guiraudon,Michael.Chu,Bob.Kiai}@lhsc.on.ca

Abstract. Traditional approaches for repairing and replacing mitral valves have relied on placing the patient on cardiopulmonary bypass (on-pump) and accessing the arrested heart directly via a median sternotomy. However, because this approach has the potential for adverse neurological, vascular and immunological sequalae, there is a push towards performing such procedures in a minimally-invasive fashion. Nevertheless, preliminary experience on animals and humans has indicated that ultrasound guidance alone is often not sufficient. This paper describes the first porcine trial of the NeoChord DS1000 (Minnetonka, MN), employed to attach neochords to a mitral valve leaflet where the traditional ultrasound guided protocol has been augmented by dynamic virtual geometric models. In addition to demonstrating that the procedure can be performed with significantly increased precision and speed (up to 6 times), we also record and compare the trajectories used by each of five surgeons to navigate the NeoChord instrument.

Keywords: Image guided surgery, mitral valve repair.

1 Introduction

Degenerative mitral valve disease (DMVD) is a common heart valve disorder where a ruptured or prolapsing valve leaflet results in incomplete mitral valve closure, often resulting in shortness of breath, fluid retention, heart failure and premature death[1]. DMVD affects 2% of the general population [2]. Severe, symptomatic disease is treated by surgical repair or replacement. DMVD is characterized by abnormal connective tissue of the mitral valve, resulting in weakening and rupture of the chordae tendonae (chords), the support structures of the mitral valve, preventing its natural closure. Major advances in mitral repair surgery have improved short- and long-term outcomes of patients with this disease [3].

Conventional open heart cardiac surgery often requires a full sternotomy, cardiopulmonary bypass, temporary cardiac arrest and is associated with longer

P. Abolmaesumi et al. (Eds.): IPCAI 2012, LNAI 7330, pp. 84–93, 2012.
© Springer-Verlag Berlin Heidelberg 2012

recovery periods, which may not be as well tolerated in elderly patients with multiple co-morbidities. Recent innovations in minimally invasive and robotic mitral repair techniques employ sternal sparing approaches to reduce the invasiveness of the procedure [4][5], but still require the use of cardiopulmonary bypass which has many associated complications. While the emerging field of transcatheter mitral valve repair avoids the risks of conventional surgery and potentially offers hopes of beating heart mitral valve reconstruction, concerns about residual mitral insufficiency, durability and inadequate mitral valve repair have been raised [6].

The NeoChord DS-1000 (NeoChord, Minnetonka, MN, USA) is a device capable of performing off-pump, mitral valve repair for certain forms of DMVD[7] [8]. The device uses trans-apical access to approach and capture the prolapsed portion of the mitral valve leaflet, attach a suture and anchor it at the apex, constraining the flail leaflet and reducing the prolapsed segment back into the left ventricle. Currently, this procedure relies exclusively on trans-oesophageal echocardiography (TEE) guidance in the form of 2D single plane, bi-plane, and 3D imaging. While TEE has thus far proven adequate for the final positioning of the tool and grasping the leaflet, there have been safety concerns relating to the navigation of the tool from the apex to the target MV leaflet. TEE guidance is problematic since it is not always possible to maintain appropriate spatial and temporal resolution in 3D, and it is not always possible using 2D and 2D bi-plane views to simultaneously maintain both the tool tip and target site in the field of view. Using 2D echo it also can be difficult to ensure that the tool tip is visualized, rather than a cross section of the tool shaft. Due to these navigation challenges, the tool can become caught in the 'subvalvar apparatus', risking chordal rupture or leaflet perforation.

Recently, a variety of augmented reality (AR) systems has been developed for intracardiac surgery [9], [10]. To improve the overall safety of the navigation process in the NeoChord procedure, we have evaluated the efficacy of employing an augmented reality technique capable of providing a robust three dimensional context for the TEE data. In this real-time environment, the surgeon can easily and intuitively identify the tool, surgical targets and high risk areas, and view tool trajectories and orientations. This paper provides a description of the overall navigation framework and proof of concept validation from an animal study. We begin with a summary of the current OR procedure workflow, followed by a discussion of our navigation system and its role in this workflow. We then describe and discuss our proof of concept experience from a porcine study.

1.1 Current OR Workflow

After extensive animal studies, the NeoChord device is currently undergoing preliminary in-human trials for the repair of flail mitral valves [11]. The procedure uses off-pump trans-apical left ventricle (LV) access. The tool is identified in 2D bi-plane echo (mitral valve commissural, mid-oesophageal long-axis view), and navigated into the commissure of the MV leaflets while the surgeon and echocardiographer attempt to maintain tool tip, tool profile, and final target

site in the echo image planes at all times. Correct position and orientation of the
tool gripper are then achieved using a 3D zoomed view. Returning to bi-plane
echo for higher temporal resolution, the prolapsing leaflet is grasped by the jaws
of the NeoChord device. Correct leaflet capture is verified using a fiber-optic
based detection mechanism. After leaflet capture has been verified, an ePTFE
(expanded polytetrafluoroethylene) suture is pulled through the leaflet and the
tool is retracted with both ends of the suture. The suture is fixed at the leaflet
with a girth hitch knot, adjusted under Doppler echo to ensure minimum mitral regurgitation (MR) and then secured at the apex using a pledget. Multiple
neochordae are typically used to ensure optimal valvular function.

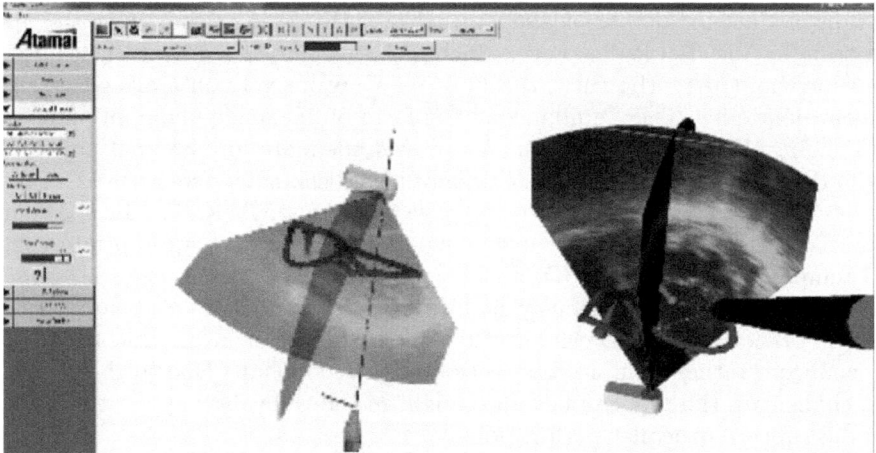

Fig. 1. Intraoperative guidance: Biplane ultrasound view augmented with targets de-
noting the Mitral (red) and Aortic (green) valve annuli, along with the representation
of the delivery device with a blue axis indicating forward trajectory and red axis indicating direction of the jaw opening. "Bullseye" view (right) shows solid echo image,
while "side" view (left) shows semi-transparent image data.

2   Methods

2.1   Augmented Echocardiography

The single largest problem in navigating the NeoChord device to the MV target
region is that echo imaging must simultaneously keep the target region (MV
line of coaptation) and the tool tip in view. To overcome this challenge, we have
developed a visualization environment [9] that uses tracking technology to locate
both the tool and the TEE probe in 3D space, making it possible to represent
the real-time echo images with virtual geometric models of both devices and
interactively defined anatomy within a common coordinate system (Fig.1). Sensors from the Aurora (Northern Digital, Waterloo, Canada) magnetic tracking

system (MTS) were integrated inside the NeoChord tool (Fig.2a) and onto the TEE probe of the Philips iE33 ultrasound (Fig.2b). Virtual geometric models of each device were created in VTK (Visualization Toolkit) and the tools appropriately calibrated [12]. Axes with 10mm markings were projected from the virtual representation of the NeoChord DS1000, indicating the forward trajectory of the tool and the direction of the opening jaws. This greatly facilitated the surgeons ability to plan their tool trajectory towards the desired target site. In addition to representations of the tools, tracking the TEE image data makes it possible to define anatomy of interest (aortic valve annulus (AVA)), target location (MV line of coaptation, and regions to be avoided (mitral valve annulus (MVA)) for contextual purposes. These geometric features are defined by the echocardiographer intraoperatively, immediately prior to the introduction of the NeoChord tool into the heart. The MVA and AVA geometries are created by manually identifying a series of tie points along each feature, and fitting a B-spline through these points. All features are identified in mid-systole, since the MV annular ring is closest to the apex at this point in the cardiac cycle. This in effect provides an indicator of the first danger zone to be avoided as the tool is moved into the left ventricle from the apex.

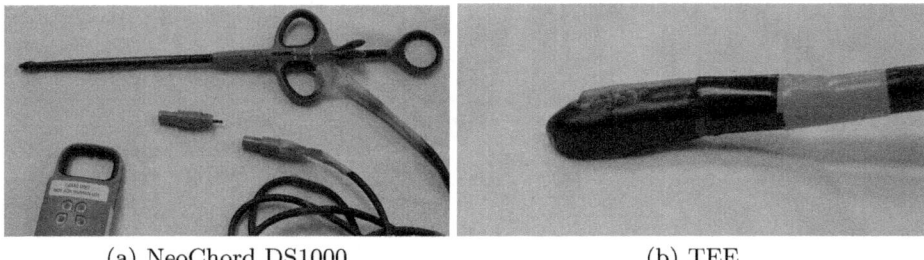

(a) NeoChord DS1000   (b) TEE

Fig. 2. Left: NeoChord DS1000 outfitted with tracking sensors. One 6-DOF sensor was installed near the tool tip, and a 5DOF sensor was built into the movable thumb grip in order to represent the tool as open or closed. Fiber-optic grasping monitor shown lower left. Right: Close-up of MTS sensor fixed to the back of the TEE transducer.

2.2   Integration into OR Workflow

Our AR guidance system is designed to assist the surgeon with three related navigation tasks; planning the left ventricular apical access point and trajectory; maintaining a safe and direct entry through the MV commisure into the left atrium, and establishing the correct tool orientation at the line of coaptation so the NeoChord DS1000 device can grasp the flail leaflet. To achieve this, prior to making the apical entry incision, the echocardiographer identifies a minimal number of tie points along the pertinent anatomy (AVA, MVA, line of coaptation). From these coordinates, a series of splines are generated to represent these features in virtual space (Fig.3a). Next, the surgeon uses the trajectory projection of the NeoChord DS1000 tool to plan the optimal entry point and orientation (Fig.3b). After apical access, the surgeon simply orients and points the tool trajectory towards the desired target site and advances the tool, monitoring the geometric model representations as seen on the real-time echo image data. By overlaying the geometric models on the real echo image data, the surgeon is able to assess the accuracy and reliability of these representations in real time. If the features have moved, for example due to the introduction of the NeoChord tool, the features can be re-defined before proceeding. Once at the desired target location, the procedure returns to the standard workflow, since additional guidance is no longer needed.

The technology associated with the AR navigation system has minimal impact in the operating room. The Aurora Tabletop magnetic field generator is specifically designed to work in the presence of various sources of metal. It has a large field of view, and easily fits on top of the OR table. Sensors attached to the TEE probe and surgical tools should not impede normal OR workflow. Furthermore, the cost associated with this technology is not prohibitive for most institutions.

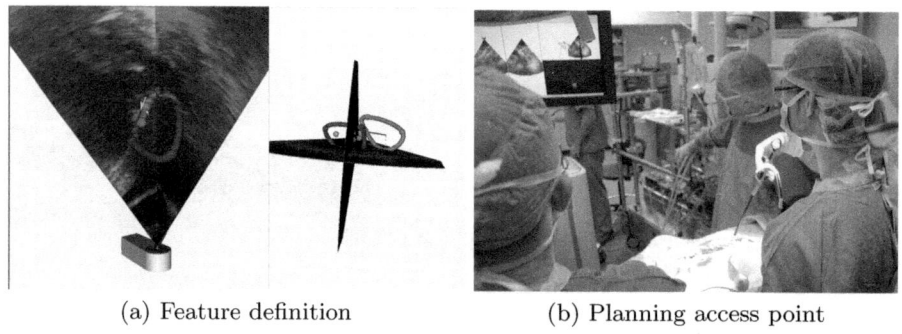

(a) Feature definition   (b) Planning access point

Fig. 3. Left: Side and 'top-down' views of intraoperatively defined anatomy (MVA in red, AVA in blue, line of coaptation in green). Right: Planning entry trajectory in the OR.

2.3   Proof of Concept: Animal Study

A porcine animal study was performed to provide a proof-of-concept validation for the AR navigation system. All procedures were performed in compliance with standards of the Ethical Review Board of Western University, London, Ontario, Canada.

A total of five cardiac surgeons participated in the study. The first goal was to evaluate different visualization options. A four-pane view showing the two bi-plane TEE images beside two AR views, which could be arbitrarily adjusted as determined by the surgeons (Fig.3b) was compared to a larger two-pane view of the AR scenes (Fig.1), with the surgeon relying on the bi-plane view on the iE33 monitor. A variety of viewing angles was evaluated anecdotally by the surgeons prior to finding a consensus. The second goal was to compare navigation of the tool from apex to target region with and without AR assistance. The surgeons were asked to navigate the NeoChord tool from a starting point near the apex, up through the mitral valve (MV) line of coaptation, situating the distal end of the tool in the left atrium. Meanwhile, the tool location was tracked and recorded at half second intervals and total navigation time was measured. The safety of the process was assessed using the tracking data, while task completion time acted as a measure of the cognitive demands placed on the surgeon.

3   Results

Prior to the study, the visualization configuration was optimized using input from the surgeons. The dual-pane AR view was consistently preferred over the four-pane version that included the bi-plane data also available on the iE33 unit. The consensus was that since the bi-plane information was readily available on an adjacent monitor, it was advantageous to have larger versions of the AR data available in the two-pane view. The surgeons quickly agreed on preferred viewing perspectives, one view representing a typical long-axis echo, the second view extending "up" from the apex towards the MVA (Fig.1). These views provided optimal intuitive presentation of navigation in all three dimensions.

Planning the point of entry at the apex and preparing the proper tool orientation was greatly facilitated by viewing the virtual tool axes relative to the MVA ring. While apical access is the standard procedure for trans-apical surgeries, there is some debate that a slightly more lateral entry point towards the papillary muscles may provide a better anchoring point for the neochordae. Our

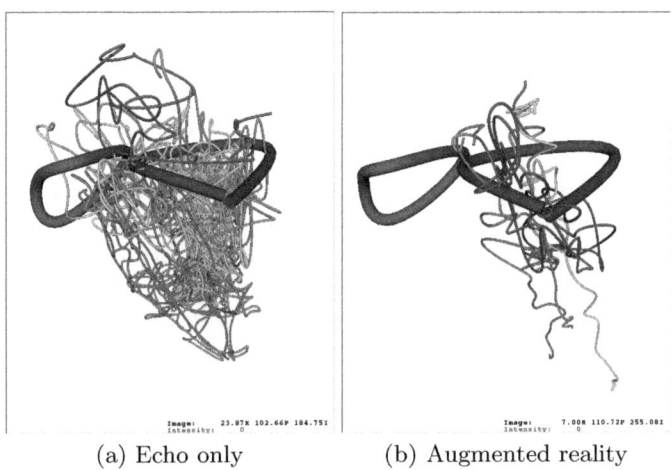

(a) Echo only   (b) Augmented reality

Fig. 4. Colour-coded tool paths for all five surgeons: AVA shown in blue, MVA in red. Left: with biplane echo guidance. Right: AR guidance.

AR navigation platform makes it possible to evaluate such questions prior to making the incision.

Magnetically tracked tool paths are shown in Figures 4a and 4b with a unique colour coding for each surgeon. Figures 5a and 5b present path data for one of the surgeons in isolation. Navigation time data are presented in Table 1.

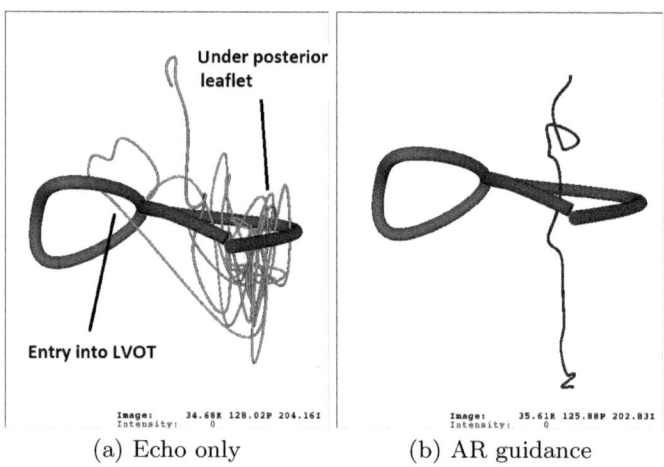

(a) Echo only   (b) AR guidance

Fig. 5. Left: Navigation path for one of the surgeons. Note entry into left ventricular outflow tract (LVOT), and getting caught under the posterior MV leaflet. Right: Same surgeon using AR guidance.

4   Discussion

Minimal AR Overlay. AR displays often add considerable information to the real visual field. While the information added may be necessary for successful guidance of a given procedure, it also invariably obscures some of the native data when the two are overlaid, as well as increases the cognitive load on the surgeon. One solution to this problem is to present the new guidance information in a separate window without any overlay onto the native data. The disadvantage of this approach is that it is difficult to identify mis-registration of preoperative or tracking data, potentially reducing procedure safety. An alternative solution is to minimize the amount of information overlaid onto the native image data. The complexity of information to present depends primarily on the surgical task and where image guidance support fits into the surgical workflow. The problem we wished to solve was the difficulty of keeping the surgical target site (MV line of coaptation) and unsafe regions (MVA), and the tool tip in the echo image plane simultaneously. Hence, the minimal data needed are the MVA at systole, (since this is it's closest approach to the tools starting point at the apex), the line of coaptation and the tool tip itself. To this we added the AVA since it provides both a helpful anatomical reference point as well as a secondary "danger zone" to avoid. Finally, the tool axes were added as a means of planning a path trajectory with minimal footprint within the visualization scene.

Intuitive Navigation. Of the five surgeons involved in the navigation test only one had previous experience using the NeoChord device, while another performed the navigation task more quickly using echo alone. The mean task completion time fell by a factor of almost six when using AR, strongly indicating the AR system greatly reduces the cognitive demands of navigating a tool using echocardiography. Previous animal studies have indicated a significant difference between expert and beginner surgeons ability to use the NeoChord device[13]. In our results, the standard deviation dropped from 94 seconds in echo-alone guidance to 8 seconds for AR navigation, suggesting the AR platform provides a more universally intuitive method for tool navigation, and can greatly reduce the learning curve associated with this surgical procedure.

Table 1. Surgeon navigation: times from apex to target site (seconds)

Surgeon	AR-enhanced echo	TEE biplane alone
1	26	264
2	15	201
3	18	92
4	35	25
5	12	36
mean	21 ± 8.3	124 ± 93.9

Safety Considerations. The graphical representation of navigation paths (Figures 4a, 4b) clearly and consistently demonstrate that more direct paths were followed during the placement of the tool in position for grasping the MV leaflet using AR navigation. Figures 5a and 5b isolate the paths taken by one surgeon (the most experienced with the device), with and without AR navigation. Two interesting phenomena can be observed in the echo-only guidance path: at one point the tool entered the left ventricular outflow tract and passed through the the aortic valve, while later it appears to be caught under the posterior MV leaflet. Both these patterns can be seen in all five echo-only datasets, while they never appear in the AR navigation paths. The phenomena of getting caught under the MV leaflet is of particular concern for this procedure, since this is the circumstance where a thin leaflet could be perforated.

Areas for Improvement. For our animal studies, two NeoChord tools were retrofitted with MTS sensors to track the tool shaft and tip locations. Sensors in both tools suffered breakdowns during the procedures and needed on-site repairs. More robust sensor integration and strain relief is planned for future work.

While our semi-automatic feature definition software provides sufficient accuracy for the procedure, it took up to 20 minutes to define the AVA, MVA and line of coaptation in systole. The line of coaptation was particularly difficult to identify in healthy porcine hearts. We believe this feature to be much easier to define in humans, particularly when a prolapsed or flailing leaflet is present.

More careful selection of standard viewing angles must be performed to permit observation of both echo image data and geometric models representing tool and anatomy; in most cases, we needed to present the echo data in a semi-transparent fashion, otherwise the geometric model elements were occluded from view. While presenting echo data in this manner did not prove to be a large problem, it is important always to rely primarily on the real ultrasound data, rather than the geometric constructs. The advantage of integrating echo with geometric model elements is that it provides real-time validation of augmented reality accuracy; when the echo image data are made semi-transparent, the surgeon's ability to verify the accuracy of geometric model elements is hampered.

5   Conclusions

We show proof-of-concept validation for augmented reality enhanced echocardiograpy intracardiac navigation for the NeoChord off-pump mitral valve repair procedure. Using echo guidance alone compared to AR navigation, five cardiac surgeons used the NeoChord device to navigate the tool from entry at the apex of the heart to a point at the line of coaptation in the mitral valve. Tracked path results clearly show improved safety and time using AR navigation.

Future work will entail improving our feature definition software, more robust sensor integration into the NeoChord, a further analysis of psychophysical factors of AR navigation, and comprehensive surgical workflow analysis to integrate AR navigation into standard of care procedures. Further animal studies are planned to provide a significant sample size for thorough comparison of AR guidance versus echo alone. In addition the visualization environment will be enhanced to integrate planning functions based on pre-operative imaging.

Acknowledgments. The authors would like to thank John Zentgraf and Arun Saini (NeoChord) for assistance with tool development, and Dr. Richard Daly (Mayo Clinic, Rochester, Minnesota) for assistance with the animal study and data analysis. Funding for this work was provided by Canadian Foundation for Innovation (20994), the Ontario Research Fund (RE-02-038) and the Canadian Institutes of Health Research (179298).

References

1. Gillinov, A.M., Cosgrove, D.M., Blackstone, E.H., Diaz, R., Arnold, J.H., Lytle, B.W., Smedira, N.G., Sabik, J.F., McCarthy, P.M., Loop, F.D.: Durability of mitral valve repair for degenerative disease. J. Thorac. Cardiovasc Surg. 116(5), 734–743 (1998)
2. Freed, L.A., Levy, D., Levine, R.A., Larson, M.G., Evans, J.C., Fuller, D.L., Lehman, B., Benjamin, E.J.: Prevalence and Clinical Outcome of Mitral-Valve Prolapse. N. Engl. J. Med. 341, 1–7 (1999)

3. Augoustides, J.G., Atluri, P.: Progress in mitral valve disease: understanding the revolution. J. Cardiothorac Vasc. Anesth. 23(6), 916–923 (2009)

4. Nifong, L.W., Chu, V.F., Bailey, B.M., Maziarz, D.M., Sorrell, V.L., Holbert, D., Chitwood Jr., W.R.: Robotic mitral valve repair: experience with the da Vinci system. Ann. Thorac. Surg. 75(2), 438–442 (2003)

5. Murphy, D.A., Miller, J.S., Langford, D.A.: Endoscopic robotic mitral valve surgery. J. Thorac. Cardiovasc. Surg. 133(4), 1119–1120 (2007); author reply 1120

6. Alfieri, O., De Bonis, M., Maisano, F., La Canna, G.: Future Directions in Degenerative Mitral Valve Repair. Seminars in Thoracic and Cardiovascular Surgery 19(2), 127–132 (2007)

7. NeoChord Inc., http://www.neochord.com/

8. Bajona, P., Katz, W.E., Daly, R.C., Kenton, J.Z., Speziali, G.: Beating-heart, off-pump mitral valve repair by implantation of artificial chordae tendineae: An acute in vivo animal study. The Journal of Thoracic and Cardiovascular Surgery, 188–193 (2009)

9. Linte, C.A., Moore, J., Wedlake, C., Bainbridge, D., Guiraudon, G.M., Jones, D.L., Peters, T.M.: Inside the beating heart: an in vivo feasibility study on fusing pre- and intra-operative imaging for minimally invasive therapy. International Journal of Computer Assisted Radiology and Surgery, 113–123 (2009)

10. Vasilyev, N.V., Novotny, P.M., Martinez, J.F., Loyola, H., Salgo, I.S., Howe, R.D., del Nido, P.J.: Stereoscopic vision display technology in real-time three-dimensional echocardiography-guided intracardiac beating-heart surgery. J. Thorac. Cardiovasc. Surg. 135(6), 1334–1341 (2008)

11. Seeburger, J., Noack, T., Lyontyev, L., Höbartner, M., Tschernich, H., Ender, J., Borger, M.A., Mohr, F.: Value of three dimensional real-time transoesophageal echocardiography in guiding transapical beating heart mitral valve repair. In: 25th EACTS Annual Meeting Interactive CardioVascular and Thoracic Surgery, S 112 (2011)

12. Gobbi, D.G., Comeau, R.M., Peters, T.M.: Ultrasound Probe Tracking for Real-Time Ultrasound/MRI Overlay and Visualization of Brain Shift. In: Taylor, C., Colchester, A. (eds.) MICCAI 1999. LNCS, vol. 1679, pp. 920–927. Springer, Heidelberg (1999)

13. Seeburger, J., Leontjev, S., Neumuth, M., Noack, T., Höbartner, M., Misfeld, M., Borger, M.A., Mohr, F.W.: Transapical beating-heart implantation of neo-chordae to mitral valve leaflets: results of an acute animal study. Eur. J. Cardiothorac. Surg. (2011)

Motion Estimation Model for Cardiac and Respiratory Motion Compensation

Sebastian Kaeppler[1], Alexander Brost[1,*], Martin Koch[1], Wen Wu[2],
Felix Bourier[3], Terrence Chen[2], Klaus Kurzidim[3],
Joachim Hornegger[1], and Norbert Strobel[4]

[1] Pattern Recognition Lab, Friedrich-Alexander-University Erlangen-Nuremberg,
Erlangen, Germany
Alexander.Brost@cs.fau.de
[2] Siemens Corporation, Corporate Research and Technology, NJ, USA
[3] Klinik für Herzrhythmusstörungen, Krankenhaus Barmherzige Brüder,
Regensburg, Germany
[4] Siemens AG, Healthcare Sector, Forchheim, Germany

Abstract. Catheter ablation is widely accepted as the best remaining
option for the treatment of atrial fibrillation if drug therapy fails. Ablation procedures can be guided by 3-D overlay images projected onto
live fluoroscopic X-ray images. These overlay images are generated from
either MR, CT or C-Arm CT volumes. As the alignment of the overlay is
often compromised by cardiac and respiratory motion, motion compensation methods are desirable. The most recent and promising approaches
use either a catheter in the coronary sinus vein, or a circumferential mapping catheter placed at the ostium of one of the pulmonary veins. As
both methods suffer from different problems, we propose a novel method
to achieve motion compensation for fluoroscopy guided cardiac ablation
procedures. Our new method localizes the coronary sinus catheter. Based
on this information, we estimate the position of the circumferential mapping catheter. As the mapping catheter is placed at the site of ablation, it provides a good surrogate for respiratory and cardiac motion. To
correlate the motion of both catheters, our method includes a training
phase in which both catheters are tracked together. The training information is then used to estimate the cardiac and respiratory motion of the
left atrium by observing the coronary sinus catheter only. The approach
yields an average 2-D estimation error of 1.99 ± 1.20 mm.

1 Introduction

An irregular fast rhythm of the left atrium - clinically described as atrial fibrillation - may cause blood clotting which bears a high risk of stroke [1]. If drug
therapy is not an option, catheter ablation is the standard treatment option [2].
Catheter ablation procedures are guided by fluoroscopic images obtained from
C-arm systems. Important targets of the ablation procedure are the ostia of the
pulmonary veins. The goal of the ablation procedure is to create a continuous

---

* Corresponding author.

P. Abolmaesumi et al. (Eds.): IPCAI 2012, LNAI 7330, pp. 94–103, 2012.
© Springer-Verlag Berlin Heidelberg 2012

lesion set around these pulmonary veins to electrically isolate them from the left atrium. In general three catheters are used during the procedure. At the beginning of the procedure, a linear catheter is placed inside the coronary sinus vein, where it is to remain fixed during the procedure. It is referred to as CS catheter. The coronary sinus vein lies between the left ventricle and the left atrium. Then, an ablation catheter and a circumferential mapping catheter are brought into the left atrium by means of two transseptal punctures. For pulmonary vein isolation, the mapping catheter is positioned at the ostium of each of the pulmonary veins (PVs) considered for ablation, in order to measure electrical signals. As the soft-tissue ablation targets inside the heart are not visible within X-ray images [3,4], overlay images generated from either CT, MR, or C-arm CT can be used during the procedures to facilitate a more accurate catheter navigation [5]. Unfortunately, the clinical value of these overlay images is reduced by cardiac and respiratory motion.

Recent approaches for motion compensation based on tracking of the CS or the circumferential mapping catheter have shown to improve the alignment of these overlay images [6,7]. The work in [6] facilitates motion compensation by using the CS catheter, whereas the method in [7] uses the circumferential mapping catheter. The downside of using the CS catheter to derive a motion estimate for animating the overlay image is due to the fact that this catheter is outside of the left atrium and close to the left ventricle. Therefore, its movement is strongly influenced by ventricular motion. This is why other authors [8] found it to be unsuitable for cardiac motion compensation in ablation procedures. The circumferential mapping catheter on the other hand has the advantage that it can be placed close to the site of ablation. In this case, the calculated catheter position can be used directly to update the overlay images. Unfortunately, relying on the mapping catheter is not without problems. For example, it may be moved on purpose during the procedure, e.g., to reposition it from one PV to another. Detecting when to stop motion compensation then either requires user interaction or a movement detection algorithm. In addition, if only one transseptal puncture is performed, only one catheter can be inside the left atrium. In this case, the circumferential mapping catheter is brought into the left atrium before and after the ablation of one PV to measure the electrical signals. Thus it may not even be avilable for motion compensation during the ablation itself. This is why we propose a new method that combines the advantage of the coronary sinus catheter, its continuous presence throughout the procedure, with the accuracy of the mapping catheter. To this end, we use a training phase during which both catheters are tracked. The acquired data is then used to set up an estimation model for the position of the mapping catheter. After that, the model can be used to estimate the cardiac and respiratory motion of the left atrium by observing the CS catheter only.

2   Motion Compensation

In order to improve the motion compensation results, we separate the motion of the CS catheter into respiratory and cardiac motion. For respiratory motion, a rigid approximation of the heart motion has shown to give good results [9]. Here, we assume that both the CS and the mapping catheter are equally affected by respiratory movement. The heart beat related motion patterns of the two catheters, however, usually differ. The displacement between the two catheters due to different cardiac motion patterns may exceed 10 mm, see Fig. 3. We use the position of the CS catheter to determine the cardiac phase of an image. Using the training data, we estimate the position of the circumferential mapping catheter based on the cardiac phase. This way we compensate for the difference in cardiac motion between the two catheters. Our method is separated into three steps. The first step is the training phase in which both the CS and the mapping catheter are tracked together. In the second step, we compute features to relate the CS catheter position to a point in the cardiac cycle. The third step is the actual live motion compensation during the procedures. The details are given in the following subsections.

2.1   Training Phase

For every image in the training phase, the circumferential mapping catheter and the CS catheter are tracked using the method proposed in [10]. The positions of the electrodes of the CS and the center of the mapping catheter are stored for later computations. The tracked electrodes of the CS catheter are denoted as $c_i^{(j)} = (u_i^{(j)}, v_i^{(j)})^T$ with $i \in \{1, 2, ..., N\}$ and N being the number of electrodes, and $j \in [1, M]$ the number of images in the training sequence. Usually, CS catheters with either four or ten electrodes are used during ablation procedures. The center of the mapping catheter in frame j is denoted as $m_j \in \mathbb{R}^2$. The image coordinate system is defined by the coordinates u and v. For simplicity, we denote the most distal electrode as c_1 and the most proximal one as c_N.

2.2   Motion Estimation Model

In order to build our model, we need to determine the cardiac phase for each training image. One could use ECG data to determine the cardiac phase for a given frame. Unfortunately, this data is not always readily available at the imaging system. Additionally, its accuracy may be affected by irregularities of the heart beat. Here, the computation of the cardiac phase is based on a pattern recognition approach instead. In particular, we exploit the fact that respiration causes only a slight rotational movement of the heart [9,11], while the electrodes of the CS catheter show a large relative rotative movement during the cardiac cycle. We try to capture this movement due to the cardiac cycle using a feature set based on the positions of the electrodes of the CS catheter. For an illustration, see Fig. 1. The following features $f_1^{(j)}, \ldots, f_5^{(j)}$ for image j are computed for all images j in the training set:

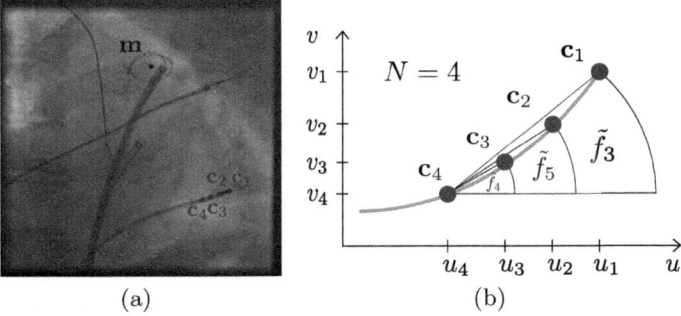

Fig. 1. Features used to calculate the cardiac cycle value μ. (a) One frame of a typical fluoroscopic sequence. (b) Illustration of the considered features.

- The first feature is the u-position of the most distal electrode divided by the u-position of the most proximal electrode. The positions are in absolute image coordinates and not related to a reference frame

$$f_1^{(j)} = u_1^{(j)}/u_N^{(j)}.\tag{1}$$

- The second feature is calculated similar to the first feature, using the v-coordinates

$$f_2^{(j)} = v_1^{(j)}/v_N^{(j)}.\tag{2}$$

- The third feature is the angle between the u-axis of the image and the line spanned by the most proximal and most distal electrode

$$f_3^{(j)} = \arctan\left(\frac{|v_1^{(j)} - v_N^{(j)}|}{|u_1^{(j)} - u_N^{(j)}|}\right).\tag{3}$$

- The fourth feature is the angle between the u-axis of the image and the line spanned by the most proximal electrode and the one next to it

$$f_4^{(j)} = \arctan\left(\frac{|v_{N-1}^{(j)} - v_N^{(j)}|}{|u_{N-1}^{(j)} - u_N^{(j)}|}\right).\tag{4}$$

- The last feature is the angle between the u-axis of the image and the line spanned by the most proximal electrode and the second next to it

$$f_5^{(j)} = \arctan\left(\frac{|v_{N-2}^{(j)} - v_N^{(j)}|}{|u_{N-2}^{(j)} - u_N^{(j)}|}\right).\tag{5}$$

These features capture CS catheter rotations and deformations, which are typical for cardiac motion. Yet, they are relatively invariant to translation motion, which is characteristically for respiratory motion. As the feature values have different

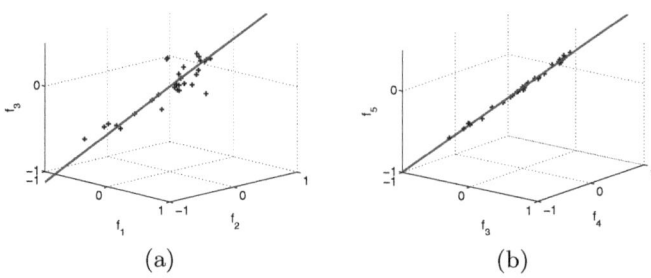

Fig. 2. Visualization of the feature space. (a) The first three features computed on the training set of sequence #12 (blue cross), and the corresponding principle axis (red line). (b) The last three features computed on the same training set, and the corresponding principle axis.

ranges, they are normalized to the range $[0, 1]$. The resulting features are denoted in vector notation as

$$\boldsymbol{f}_j = (\tilde{f}_1^{(j)}, \tilde{f}_2^{(j)}, \tilde{f}_3^{(j)}, \tilde{f}_4^{(j)}, \tilde{f}_5^{(j)})^T. \tag{6}$$

To reduce the dimensionality of the feature vector, a principle component analysis is performed. First, the mean feature vector is calculated by

$$\bar{\boldsymbol{f}} = \frac{1}{M} \sum_{j=1}^{M} \boldsymbol{f}_j. \tag{7}$$

In the next step, the covariance matrix is calculated by

$$\boldsymbol{\Sigma} = \frac{1}{M-1} \sum_{j=1}^{M} (\boldsymbol{f}_j - \bar{\boldsymbol{f}}) \cdot (\boldsymbol{f}_j - \bar{\boldsymbol{f}})^T. \tag{8}$$

Now, the eigenvalues and eigenvectors of $\boldsymbol{\Sigma}$ are computed. Let $\boldsymbol{e}_\lambda$ be the eigenvector corresponding to the largest eigenvalue of the covariance matrix $\boldsymbol{\Sigma}$. The unitless cardiac cycle value μ_j for every image in the training sequence is finally computed by

$$\mu_j = \boldsymbol{e}_\lambda^T \cdot (\boldsymbol{f}_j - \bar{\boldsymbol{f}}), \tag{9}$$

which is the length of the orthogonal projection of the feature vector onto the first eigenvector. Fig. 2 shows the fit of $\boldsymbol{e}_\lambda$ to the features in feature space. Thus, a correspondence between the calculated cardiac cycle value μ_j and the stored position of the mapping catheter $\boldsymbol{m}_j$ has been established: $\mu_j \rightarrow \boldsymbol{m}_j$. One example of the relationship between μ and the intracardiac motion is depicted in Fig. 3.

2.3 Motion Compensation

For motion compensation, only the tracking results for the CS catheter are required. To apply the compensation, the feature vector needs to be computed for the new image. This feature vector $\boldsymbol{f}_{\text{new}}$ is calculated from the tracked CS catheter position as described above. The new cycle value is calculated by

$$\mu_{\text{new}} = \boldsymbol{e}_{\lambda}^{T} \cdot (\boldsymbol{f}_{\text{new}} - \bar{\boldsymbol{f}}). \tag{10}$$

In the next step of the motion compensation, two training samples that are closest to the current image with respect to cardiac phase need to be found. The first one, denoted β, is earlier in the cardiac cycle than the new image. The other one, denoted γ, is later. To do so, the following minimization problem is considered for the sample index β:

$$\beta = \underset{j}{\arg\min}(1 + |\mu_j - \mu_{\text{new}}|)^2 + \alpha \cdot (u_N^{(j)} - u_N^{(\text{new})})^2. \tag{11}$$
$$\scriptstyle \mu_j < \mu_{\text{new}}$$

For the sample γ, the constraint $\mu_j < \mu_{new}$ in Eq. (11) is replaced by $\mu_j \geq \mu_{new}$. The position of the most proximal electrode in u-direction, $u_N^{(\text{new})}$, is used for regularization. The idea behind this term is to reduce the effect of errors in the calculation of the heart cycle, which may, for example, arrise from slight inaccuracies in the catheter tracking. The cardiac cycle values μ_β and μ_γ correspond to the two samples closest to the new frame with the observed cardiac cycle value μ_{new}. Using these two values, two estimates for the position of the circumferential mapping catheter are computed as

$$\hat{\boldsymbol{m}}_{\text{new},\beta} = \boldsymbol{m}_\beta + \left(\boldsymbol{c}_N^{(\text{new})} - \boldsymbol{c}_N^{(\beta)} \right), \tag{12}$$

$$\hat{\boldsymbol{m}}_{\text{new},\gamma} = \boldsymbol{m}_\gamma + \left(\boldsymbol{c}_N^{(\text{new})} - \boldsymbol{c}_N^{(\gamma)} \right). \tag{13}$$

The difference terms in Eqs. (12, 13) provide the compensation for respiratory motion. For two images in the same cardiac phase, we assume that any remaining motion must be due to respiration. Since we also assume that the CS and the mapping catheter are equally affected by respiratory motion, we simply apply the difference vector between the proximal electrodes of the CS catheter in the two images to the estimate of the position of the mapping catheter. The proximal electrode was chosen because it shows the least intracardiac motion w.r.t. the mapping catheter. These two values are combined to calculate the final estimate as

$$\hat{\boldsymbol{m}}_{\text{new}} = \phi \cdot \hat{\boldsymbol{m}}_{\text{new},\beta} + (1 - \phi) \cdot \hat{\boldsymbol{m}}_{\text{new},\gamma}. \tag{14}$$

The scaling value ϕ between the two estimates is calculated by

$$\phi = \frac{|\mu_\gamma - \mu_{\text{new}}|}{|\mu_\gamma - \mu_\beta|}. \tag{15}$$

In case of high acquisition frame rates ≥ 15 frames-per-second, we apply a temporal lowpass filter

$$\hat{\boldsymbol{m}}'_{\text{new}} = \delta \cdot \hat{\boldsymbol{m}}_{\text{new}} + (1 - \delta) \cdot \hat{\boldsymbol{m}}_{\text{new}-1}. \tag{16}$$

This is motivated by the fact that the motion of the heart is smooth in high frame rate image sequences.

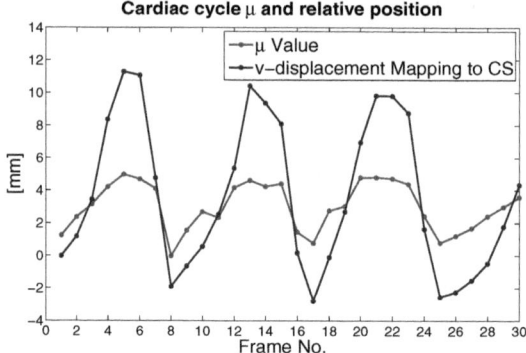

Fig. 3. Calculated μ values for a training set and the displacement between the proximal electrode of the CS and the center of the mapping catheter in v-direction [mm], w.r.t. a reference frame

3   Evaluation and Results

For evaluation, 13 fluoroscopy sequences from three different hospitals were used[1]. The length of the sequences varied between 47 and 150 frames, or two to 47 seconds. Each sequence was split into two disjoint sets of frames. One set, comprising the first 30 frames of the sequence, was used for the patient-specific training of the model. The remaining set was used for evaluation. This resulted in a total number of 958 frames available for evaluation. In a clinical scenario, usually more time passes between training and compensation phase. An evaluation with a simulated clinical workflow is subject of further research. The first sequence was acquired using ECG-triggered fluoroscopy. We chose to include this sequence to see how our method handles respiratory motion with only residual cardiac motion. The other sequences were acquired with either 15 or 30 frames-per-second. We compare our results to an uncompensated overlay as well as to the reference method proposed in [6]. The error is defined as the 2-D Euclidean distance between the estimated position of the overlay, determined by the motion compensation algorithm, and the center of the mapping catheter. Due to its proximity to the ablation target, the motion of the mapping catheter is considered to be the motion that needs to be estimated. For an illustration, see Fig. 5. The values of 0.01 for regularization parameter α and 0.7 for the smoothing parameter δ were determined by performing a grid search on a subsample of the available sequences. The results for the individual sequences are given in Fig. 4. On our available data set, the observed motion was 3.59 mm $\pm$ 2.27 mm. The reference method, proposed in [6,12], yielded an error of 4.65 mm $\pm$ 3.33 mm, which, surprisingly, is higher than the observed motion. Our new approach incorporating the estimation model yielded a compensation error of 1.98 mm $\pm$ 1.30 mm.

---

[1] The data are available from the authors upon request for non-commercial research.

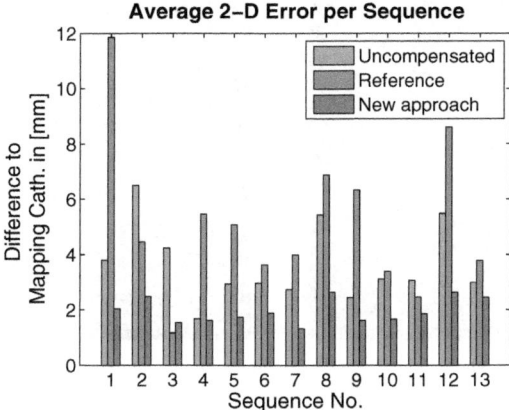

Fig. 4. The results for our motion compensation approach, compared to the reference method in [6], and the misalignment error for an uncompensated approach

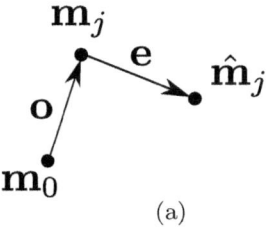

Frames	Avg. Error [mm]
Uncomp.	3.65 ± 2.36
10	2.87 ± 2.06
20	2.61 ± 1.86
30	2.10 ± 1.35
40	2.01 ± 1.37
50	1.93 ± 1.32

(a)   (b)

Fig. 5. Error definition and varying number of training frames. (a) The observed motion o and the estimation error e in frame j. (b) Average error with varying number of training frames. A subset of the complete evaulation set, comprising 701 frames was used to calculate the average error.

4   Discussion and Conclusions

For our datasets, the proposed method has outperformed the reference motion compensation approach proposed in [6,12]. We believe that this is due to the fact that our data was acquired with different X-ray acquisition settings, either regarding frame rate, C-arm position, or both. We also point out that we measured the error on the X-ray detector, whereas in [6,12], it was measured at the iso-center of the C-arm coordinate system. Due to the magnification involved in perspective projection, our error appears larger. Unfortunately, the data used in [6,12] was not available for comparison. The reference method uses a Butterworth low-pass filter to smooth the cardiac motion of the CS catheter and directly applies this motion to the overlay. This approach relies on the assumption that both the CS and the left atrium move in sync, with the CS catheter experiencing a higher amount of cardiac motion compared to the mapping catheter.

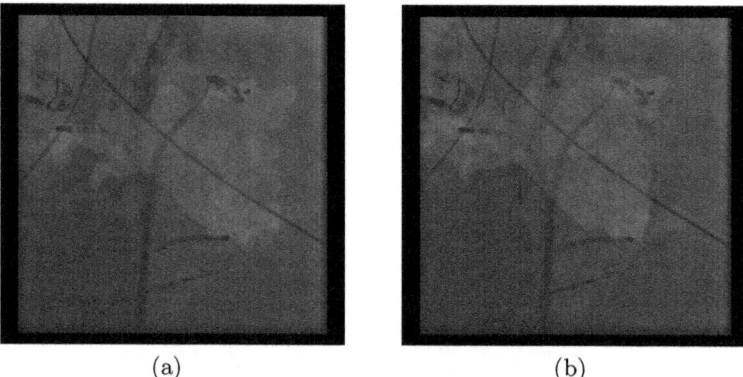

(a)   (b)

Fig. 6. A comparison showing the difference if motion compensation is considered or not. (a) One frame without motion compensation. (b) Shows the same frame as in (a), but this time with motion compensation. Best viewed in color.

Another assumption required is that their respective motion directions are the same. The application of a suitably designed lowpass filter can then reduce the amplitude of the cardiac motion estimated from the CS catheter to the amplitude of the cardiac motion of the mapping catheter. Unfortunately, on our data set, these assumptions are not always valid, explaining the higher errors of the reference method. Other researchers also found that the CS and the left atrium need not always follow the same motion pattern [8]. Our estimation model does not depend on these assumptions. In addition, our method does not require older frames for low-pass filtering, making it suitable for low acquisition frame rates. Experiments have shown that about thirty frames are sufficient for the training of our model, see Fig. 5. As expected, both approaches perform not as well as the approach involving the direct tracking of the circumferential mapping catheter [13]. Since the error of our method is still higher than when using the mapping catheter directly, a combination of both methods should be considered. Recent work in [7] already utilized the CS catheter to detect non-physiological movement of the circumferential mapping catheter. In such a case, we may want to switch to CS catheter based motion estimation. Since the currently proposed method deals only with 2-D images, it is prone to suffer from foreshortening which can be difficult to detect in monoplane images. Fortunately, out of plane motion primarily affects the size of the 3-D overlay, and size changes of the left atrium are much less relevant than discrepancies due to heart and breathing motion. The proposed method could be extended to 3-D compensation by performing the training in biplane mode. This way one could estimate 3-D motion while observing 2-D motion. The current implementation of our motion compensation approach achieves about 20 fps. Most of the time per frame is required for catheter tracking. The motion estimation model is calculated within 50 ms. The estimation of the mapping catheter position using the proposed model is performed in less than 10 ms. An example of our motion compensation approach is shown in Fig. 6.

References

1. Wolf, P., Abbott, R., Kannel, W.: Atrial fibrillation as an independent risk factor for stroke: the framingham study. Stroke 22, 983–988 (1991)
2. Cappato, R., Calkins, H., Chen, S.A., Davies, W., Iesaka, Y., Kalman, J., Kim, Y.H., Klein, G., Packer, D., Skanes, A.: Worldwide survey on the methods, efficacy, and safety of catheter ablation for human atrial fibrillation. Circulation 111, 1100–1105 (2005)
3. Prümmer, M., Hornegger, J., Lauritsch, G., Wigström, L., Girard-Hughes, E., Fahrig, R.: Cardiac C-arm CT: a unified framework for motion estimation and dynamic CT. IEEE Transact. Med. Imaging 28(11), 1836–1849 (2009)
4. Strobel, N., Meissner, O., Boese, J., Brunner, T., Heigl, B., Hoheisel, M., Lauritsch, G., Nagel, M., Pfister, M., Rührnschopf, E.-P., Scholz, B., Schreiber, B., Spahn, M., Zellerhoff, M., Klingenbeck-Regn, K.: Imaging with Flat-Detector C-Arm Systems. In: Reiser, M.F., Becker, C.R., Nikolaou, K., Glazer, G. (eds.) Multislice CT (Medical Radiology / Diagnostic Imaging), 3rd edn., pp. 33–51. Springer, Heidelberg (2009)
5. De Buck, S., Maes, F., Ector, J., Bogaert, J., Dymarkowski, S., Heidbüchel, H., Suetens, P.: An Augmented Reality System for Patient-Specific Guidance of Cardiac Catheter Ablation Procedures. IEEE Transact. Med. Imaging 24(11), 1512–1524 (2005)
6. Ma, Y., King, A.P., Gogin, N., Rinaldi, C.A., Gill, J., Razavi, R., Rhode, K.S.: Real-Time Respiratory Motion Correction for Cardiac Electrophysiology Procedures Using Image-Based Coronary Sinus Catheter Tracking. In: Jiang, T., Navab, N., Pluim, J.P.W., Viergever, M.A. (eds.) MICCAI 2010. LNCS, vol. 6361, pp. 391–399. Springer, Heidelberg (2010)
7. Brost, A., Wu, W., Koch, M., Wimmer, A., Chen, T., Liao, R., Hornegger, J., Strobel, N.: Combined Cardiac and Respiratory Motion Compensation for Atrial Fibrillation Ablation Procedures. In: Fichtinger, G., Martel, A., Peters, T. (eds.) MICCAI 2011, Part I. LNCS, vol. 6891, pp. 540–547. Springer, Heidelberg (2011)
8. Klemm, H., Steven, D., Johnsen, C., Ventura, R., Rostock, T., Lutomsky, B., Risius, T., Meinertz, T., Willems, S.: Catheter motion during atrial ablation due to the beating heart and respiration: impact on accuracy and spatial referencing in three-dimensional mapping. Heart Rhythm 4(5), 587–592 (2007)
9. McLeish, K., Hill, D., Atkinson, D., Blackall, J., Razavi, R.: A study of the motion and deformation of the heart due to respiration. IEEE Transact. Med. Imaging 21(9), 1142–1150 (2002)
10. Wu, W., Chen, T., Barbu, A., Wang, P., Strobel, N., Zhou, S., Comaniciu, D.: Learning-based hypothesis fusion for robust catheter tracking in 2D X-ray fluoroscopy. In: IEEE Conference on Computer Vision and Pattern Recognition (CVPR 2011), pp. 1097–1104 (2011)
11. Shechter, G., Ozturk, C., Resar, J., McVeigh, E.: Respiratory motion of the heart from free breathing coronary angiograms. IEEE Transact. Med. Imaging 23(8), 1046–1056 (2004)
12. Ma, Y., King, A., Gogin, N., Gijsbers, G., Rinaldi, C., Gill, J., Razavi, R., Rhode, K.: Clinical evaluation of respiratory motion compensation for anatomical roadmap guided cardiac electrophysiology procedures. IEEE Transact. Biomed. Engineering (2011); Epub ahead of print
13. Brost, A., Liao, R., Hornegger, J., Strobel, N.: Model-based registration for motion compensation during EP ablation procedures. In: Fischer, B., Dawant, B., Lorenz, C. (eds.) WBIR 2010. LNCS, vol. 6204, pp. 234–245. Springer, Heidelberg (2010)

Cardiac Unfold: A Novel Technique for Image-Guided Cardiac Catheterization Procedures

YingLiang Ma[1], Rashed Karim[1], R. James Housden[1], Geert Gijsbers[2],
Roland Bullens[2], Christopher Aldo Rinaldi[3], Reza Razavi[1],
Tobias Schaeffter[1], and Kawal S. Rhode[1]

[1] Division of Imaging Sciences and Biomedical Engineering, King's College London,
SE1 7EH, UK
[2] Interventional X-ray, Philips Healthcare, Best, The Netherlands
[3] Department of Cardiology, Guy's & St. Thomas' Hospitals NHS Foundation Trust,
London, SE1 7EH, UK
y.ma@kcl.ac.uk

Abstract. X-ray fluoroscopically-guided cardiac catheterization procedures are commonly carried out for the treatment of cardiac arrhythmias, such as atrial fibrillation (AF) and cardiac resynchronization therapy (CRT). X-ray images have poor soft tissue contrast and, for this reason, overlay of a 3D roadmap derived from pre-procedure volumetric image data can be used to add anatomical information. However, current overlay technologies have the limitation that 3D information is displayed on a 2D screen. Therefore, it is not possible for the cardiologist to appreciate the true positional relationship between anatomical/functional data and the position of the interventional devices. We prose a navigation methodology, called *cardiac unfold*, where an entire cardiac chamber is unfolded from 3D to 2D along with all relevant anatomical and functional information and coupled to real-time device tracking. This would allow more intuitive navigation since the entire 3D scene is displayed simultaneously on a 2D plot. A real-time unfold guidance platform for CRT was developed, where navigation is performed using the standard AHA 16-segment bull's-eye plot for the left ventricle (LV). The accuracy of the unfold navigation was assessed in 13 patient data sets by computing the registration errors of the LV pacing lead electrodes and was found to be 2.2 ± 0.9 mm. An unfold method was also developed for the left atrium (LA) using trimmed B-spline surfaces. The method was applied to 5 patient data sets and its utility was demonstrated for displaying information from delayed enhancement MRI of patients that had undergone radio-frequency ablation.

1   Introduction

Minimally-invasive catheter-based interventions have become the treatment of choice for patients with many forms of cardiovascular disease. The cardiac catheterization laboratory is the primary treatment environment for these procedures and X-ray fluoroscopy is the main imaging modality that is used for interventional guidance. Interventional devices, such as catheters, have been specifically designed to be

P. Abolmaesumi et al. (Eds.): IPCAI 2012, LNAI 7330, pp. 104–114, 2012.

highly-visible using fluoroscopy. However, navigation can be difficult because the target structures, such as the cardiac chambers and the great vessels, are not well-visualized using fluoroscopy without the use of repeated contrast agent injection. Long procedure times, high radiation dose and large contrast agent burden have lead to the introduction of image-guided navigation solutions. The use of this technology is exemplified in the case of electrophysiology (EP) procedures and cardiac resynchronization therapy (CRT). Examples of such technology include the EnSite Velocity (St. Jude Medical, USA), CARTO 3 (Biosense Webster, USA) and EP Navigator (Philips Healthcare, The Netherlands) systems. In each of these systems, three-dimensional (3D) anatomical models of the target cardiac chambers are used to guide the interventions. In the case of EnSite Velocity and CARTO 3, these models are reconstructed using tracked catheters that are moved inside the target chamber to generate the anatomy. In the case of EP Navigator, pre-procedural computer tomography [1], magnetic resonance imaging (MRI) [2], or rotational X-ray angiography [3, 4] of the heart are used to generate the anatomical models which are then registered to and overlaid onto X-ray fluoroscopy to provide a roadmap image.

Recently, the use of cardiac MRI to guide cardiac resynchronization therapy (CRT) for patients with heart failure has been proposed and demonstrated [5-7]. CRT involves the placement of a pacemaker device with pacing leads being inserted endocardially into the right atrium (RA) and right ventricle (RV), and epicardially into the left ventricle (LV) through the coronary venous system. There is potential to reduce the high failure rate (30%) of this procedure using advanced image-guidance. Cardiac MRI can be used to obtain all the critical information necessary for successful lead placement during CRT: (a) cardiac chamber anatomy; (b) coronary venous anatomy; (c) ventricular scar distribution; and (d) dyssynchrony information. Using a prototype version of the EP Navigator, we were previously able to place the LV pacing lead to target pre-selected segments of the LV based on the MRI information [5, 6].

One limitation of current navigation approaches is that the critical information required by the cardiologist for navigation is always displayed as a projection from 3D to 2D, i.e. on the computer display screen. In the case of anatomical overlay systems, such as EP Navigator, this means that the relationship between the position of interventional devices, such as the pacing leads, and the anatomical and functional information in the roadmap cannot easily be appreciated. In the case of electroanatomical mapping systems, such as EnSite Velocity or CARTO 3, there is frequent need to rotate the 3D anatomical models to obtain the correct view.

One way to overcome this limitation is to unfold the 3D information to 2D, something that has been applied extensively for the brain [8]. 2D representation of the LV using the American Heart Association (AHA) 16-segment bull's-eye plot is a well-established technique. Furthermore, it has been shown how additional information can be added to this. For example, Termeer et al. [9] presented combination of the coronary artery centreline and scar information on a bull's-eye plot. In this paper, this concept is extended for the use of interventional guidance by coupling the bull's-eye representation with real-time device tracking. A complete unfold guidance platform was developed for specific guidance of CRT procedures. Secondly, in order to extend the unfold concept for the guidance of radio-frequency ablation of atrial fibrillation, an unfold method for the left atrium (LA) surface was developed using trimmed B-spline surfaces. These unfolding techniques, termed *cardiac unfold*, were applied to patient data: 13 data sets from patients undergoing CRT were used for off-line accuracy validation of the LV unfolding and real-time testing of the augmented navigation approach was used in 5 live CRT cases; for LA unfolding, only proof-of-concept is presented using 5 data sets from patients that underwent radiofrequency ablation for atrial fibrillation.

2   LV Unfolding Method

Cardiac MRI (Philips 1.5T Achieva, Phillips Healthcare, Best, The Netherlands) was performed prior to the pacemaker implants for 18 patients being treated for heart failure using CRT. Cardiac MRI consisted of a combination of anatomical and functional scans such as steady-state-free-precession (SSFP) and delayed enhancement (DE) scans. 3D SSFP whole-heart image data was automatically segmented to yield the endocardial surfaces of the RV, LA and RA and the endocardial and epicardial surfaces of the LV using a model-based segmentation algorithm [10]. The coronary veins and any myocardial scar were segmented from the MR images and dyssynchrony was quantified (see [6] for further details). Then the unfolding is carried out using the following methods:

2.1   3D to 2D Bull's-Eye Transformation

A transformation was designed to map the 3D anatomical/functional information to a 2D bull's-eye plot based on the standard AHA 16-segment model of the LV. An automatic method was designed using only the LV and RV surfaces which are extracted from the automatic segmentation results. A cubic Bezier curve is used to model the LV long axis. The cubic Bezier curve is defined as:

$$B(t) = (1-t)^3 P_0 + 3t(t-1)^2 P_1 + 3t^2(1-t)P_2 + t^3 P_3 \qquad t \in [0,1] \tag{1}$$

where P_i are the control points. P_0 is the apex of the LV. P_1, P_2 and P_3 are the center points of cross sections perpendicular to the long axis. To search for the locations of the control points of the Bezier curve, the following 4 steps were used: Step (1): use the automatic whole-heart segmentation algorithm to segment the LV and RV from the whole-heart MRI data and extract the LV and RV surfaces using the marching cubes algorithm; Step (2): use a linear regression algorithm to calculate the principal axis of the LV surface (figure 1A). The principal axis is defined as the first eigenvector of the positive definite matrix M_{pd}, where $M_{pd} = (1/n)A^T A$. n is the number of vertices in the LV surface. Matrix A is defined as $A = V - \overline{V}$, where V is the vertex array of the LV surface and $\overline{V}$ is the mean of all vertices; Step (3): project all vertices of the LV surface to the principle axis and find the lowest vertex. The lowest vertex is used as the apex of the LV; Step (4): calculate the center points of cross sections.

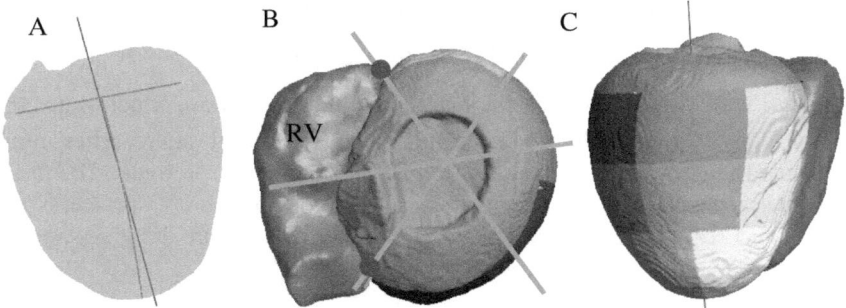

Fig. 1. (A) Principal axes (red lines) of the LV. The center Bezier curve (green curve). (B) Two landmarks (red spots) are used to divide the circular section into 6 segments. (C) Final result of automatic LV subdivision method.

After construction of the Bezier curve, it is used as the center curve of the LV surface (see figure 1A). The next step is to map all 3D vertices of the LV to the 2D bull's-eye plot. Similar to the standard LV subdivision method, two landmarks of each circular section are identified automatically by searching the attachment points of the RV to the LV (see figure 1B). This can be done in two steps: Step (1): calculate a line on the circular section from the center of the RV cross section to the center of the LV circular section; Step (2): use the line calculated in Step (1) as the reference line and search for the RV vertex in the RV cross section that forms the maximum angle between the reference line and the line from the RV vertex to the center of the LV circular section. Now, for any vertex on the LV surface, we can calculate its projection point on the center Bezier curve and obtain a parameter t in the curve function $B(t)$. It can be used as the radius in the polar coordinate system (bull's-eye plot). The angle θ between the line from this vertex to the center of the circular section and the reference line can be used as the angle in the polar coordinate system. However, using the landmarks on the RV surface boundary will not always create 6 equal subdivisions of a full circle (each division should be $60°$ in the bull's-eye plot). Therefore, a linear warp function $W(\theta)$ is used to map the angle θ in the LV surface to the angle $W(\theta)$ used in the polar coordinate system. Finally, any 3D vertex $P(x, y, z)$ on the LV surface can be transformed into a 2D point $B(t, W(\theta))$ in the polar coordinate system. Figure 1C demonstrates the final result of our method.

2.2   Mapping 3D Coronary Sinus and Scar into 2D Bull's-Eye Plot

The coronary sinus (CS) is one of the key structures for CRT guidance. The 3D vertices on the CS model can be mapped into 2D by using the same transformation for mapping the LV surface. However, when mapping into 2D, the coronary vein triangulation topology will be lost. To re-triangulate the mapped 2D points, an unconstrained Delaunay triangulation was used (see figure 2A). Each triangle in the Delaunay triangulation is labeled as inside or outside based on the edge length rule

[11]. The edge length rule labels any triangle with any of its edges larger than a threshold as outside. The threshold is set to $\sqrt{3}$ times the voxel size in the 3D MR image. $\sqrt{3}$ was chosen based on the marching cubes algorithm, which states that the longest edge of a triangle is the diagonal of the voxel cube. After removing the outside triangles, the 2D model of the CS is generated (see figure 2B). Next, the binarized scar map, which represents the scar locations on the LV surface, is mapped into 2D. The 2D representation of scar is as a 2D mesh. Figure 2C gives an example of 2D representations of the CS and scar map.

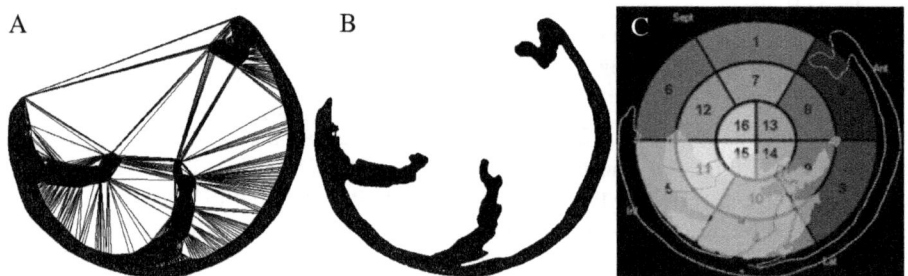

Fig. 2. (A) 2D Delaunay triangulation. (B) After removing the outside triangles. (C) The 2D bull's-eye plot with the CS (blue lines) and scar (transparent white mesh).

3   LA Unfolding Method

MR imaging was performed on 5 patients (mean age 60±10, 4 male) after radiofrequency ablation treatment for treatment of paroxysmal atrial fibrillation. This included Gadolinium-enhanced MR angiography (MRA) and DE imaging. The LA was automatically segmented from the MRA data using [12] followed by manual corrections by a clinical expert, when required. The LA surface was unfolded using the following steps:

3.1   Generation of B-Spline Contours

B-spline contours are obtained by scanning the LA segmentation in a raster-like fashion (see figure 3A) in the head-to-foot direction. Each scan line generates a contour. It is ensured that no multiple disjoint contours are generated for a single scan line. This can be a problem especially if the pulmonary veins (PVs) are not truncated at the ostium (see PV cut planes in figure 3A). Thus by carefully selecting appropriate cut planes to remove each pulmonary vein, each scan line only generates a single contour. For each contour, a distance-minimizing B-spline curve with 100 control points is then fitted through points sampled on the contour. B-spline curve fitting of these contours is important as it significantly reduces the noise within contour points.

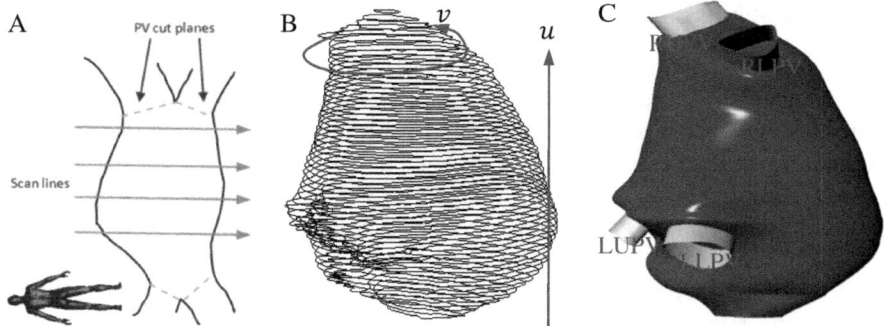

Fig. 3. (A) The generation of B-spline contours using scan lines. The human figure in the bottom-left indicates LA orientation. (B) B-spline curve contours. Arrows demonstrate the directions of u and v parameters. (C) B-spline surface constructed from the contours. Four cut-off PVs have been added for illustration purposes. (LUPV is left upper PV. LLPV is left lower PV. RUPV is right upper PV. RLPV is right lower PV).

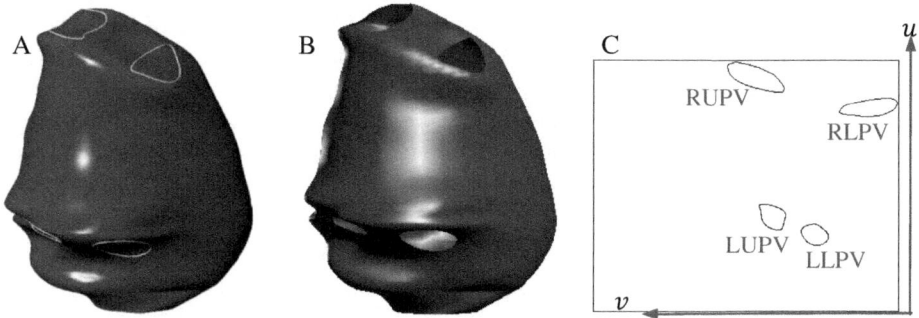

Fig. 4. (A) The LA surface with trimming curves. (B) The trimmed LA surface. (C) 2D uv map of the B-spline surface with 4 mapped trimmed curves.

3.2   Construction of B-Spline LA Model

A cubic B-spline surface is used to fit the main body of the LA from which 4 PVs have been cut and it is defined as $S(u,v) = \sum_{i=0}^{n}\sum_{j=0}^{m} N_{i,3}(u)N_{j,3}(v)P_{i,j}$. Where $\{P_{i,j}\}$ are the control points and $0 \leq u,v \leq 1$. $N_{i,3}(u)$ and $N_{j,3}(u)$ are cubic B-spline basis functions defined on the knot vector $U = \{u_0, u_1, \ldots, u_{n+3+1}\}$ and $V = \{v_0, v_1, \ldots, v_{m+3+1}\}$. The control point net $\{P_{i,j}\}$ is constructed from the control points of the B-spline curve contours. After the surface is constructed, it is rebuilt by undersampling the control points so that a smooth LA surface is created (see figure 3C). The rebuilt surface has 20x10 control points. Then 4 B-spline curves around the PV cutting regions are projected onto the B-spline surface to create 4 trimming curves (see figure 4A). The B-spline surface is trimmed in the region of the PVs using the trimming curves. The final result is shown in figure 4B.

3.3   Unfolding LA Surface into 2D Warped Parametric Map

The trimmed B-spline surface is first unfolded into the 2D parametric map (see figure 4C), which is generated after the trimmed surface is constructed. With the B-spline surface defined on (u, v) parameters, the 3D surface is naturally unfolded into the 2D parametric map. The linearity between the 3D surface and the 2D parametric map needs to be improved, so that the surface distance on the LA between any pair of points is proportional to the distance between their mapped pairs on the 2D map. To achieve this, the 2D parametric map is warped along the directions of u and v. As the LA B-spline surface is constructed from a series of evenly spaced 2D contours and u is set as the direction along the contour level direction (see figure 3B), the distance traveled along the u direction is linear. On the other hand, as contours at different levels have different lengths and the v direction is set as the circular direction around the contours (see figure 3B), the distance traveled along the v direction is non-linear. Therefore, the 2D parametric map needs to be warped along the v direction to restore the linearity.

To warp the map, we first cut the trimmed B-spline surface at the iso-line ($v = 0.5$). The iso-line is defined by the points that have constant u or v values. The lengths of the iso-line segment ($0 \leq v \leq 0.5$) and the iso-line segment ($0.5 \leq v \leq 1.0$) at the evenly spaced u levels (see figure 5A) are calculated and the 2D parametric map is warped along the v direction according to the lengths of the iso-line segmentation (see figure 5B). In order to maintain the same length ratio between u and v, the 2D parametric map is also scaled along the u direction so that the length along the u direction is equal to the length along the v direction. The final result with the trimming curves is shown in figure 5C.

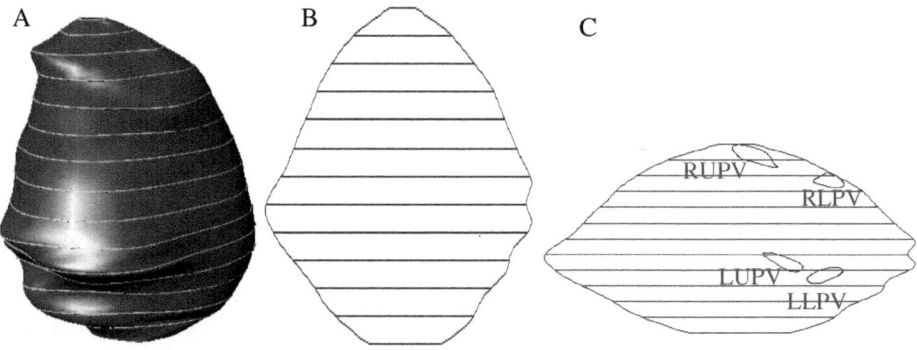

Fig. 5. (A) The iso-line segments at the evenly spaced u levels. (B) The 2D parametric map warped along the v direction. (C) The final result with trimming curves.

4   Results

4.1   The Accuracy of LV Unfolding Navigation

Unlike the LA surface unfolding, the LV surface unfolding method directly uses the LV mesh and transfers to 2D polar coordinates. Therefore, there are no model or surface fitting errors. Instead, we investigated the navigation accuracy using the LV unfolding method. 13 datasets from 13 patients were used for off-line validation. The MR data was of sufficient quality to allow the generation of the coronary venous system including the main three sub-branches. The models were registered successfully to the X-ray fluoroscopic data in all cases. The details of the registration method can be found in [6]. The respiratory motion was compensated by tracking the diaphragm in the X-ray images [13]. The registration errors in the 2D bull's-eye plot were calculated as the mean distance between the 2D pacing lead electrode positions (see crosses in figure 6) and the center curve of the CS sub-branches. The mapped lead position is automatically calculated and the centreline is manually defined. The measured error is the total error in the navigation system and encompasses all steps from segmentation to unfolding and registration to device tracking. An accuracy of 2.2 ± 0.9 mm was achieved for 602 X-ray fluoroscopic images from the 13 cases. The pixel to mm transformation was achieved by using the radius of the bull's-eye plot. In the 3D anatomical model derived from MR data, the radius corresponds to the distance from the apex to the center of the mitral valve along the long axis of the LV. Therefore, a ratio between the pixel size in the 2D bull's-eye plot and mm in the 3D anatomical model can be calculated.

For the real-time testing of the unfold guidance in 5 clinical cases, the 2D bull's-eye guidance platform was able to record and display different LV lead pacing positions both in the 3D overlay view and in the 2D bull's-eye view together with the dyssynchrony color map. The clinician was able to successfully place the pacing lead in the targeted LV segment with adequate pacing thresholds.

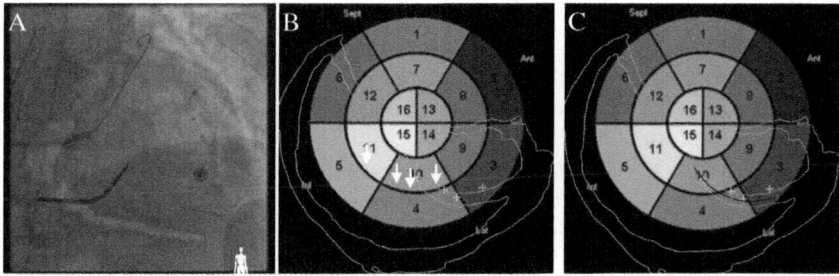

Fig. 6. (A) Overlay of the LV and CS onto an X-ray image. The blue sphere is the position of the lead electrode. (B) 2D unfolding navigation screenshot. The light blue contour is the CS tree unfolded in the 2D bull's-eye plot. The white crosses are the positions of the pacing leads. (C) Screenshot with the manual annotation of the centerline of the CS sub-branch (the dark blue line).

4.2   LA Unfolding Accuracy

To test the accuracy of the LA surface unfolding, 5 patient datasets were used (patient mean age 60 ± 10, 4 male and 1 female). Since we have only reached the unfolding stage for the LA, the only measure of error that we can currently quote is the surface fitting error as the initial B-spline surface fitting is an approximation. The surface fitting error is the Euclidean distance error between the vertices on the LA mesh which is directly extracted from the LA segmentation result (after removing 4 PVs) and projected points on the B-spline surface. An overall error of 0.8 ± 0.8 mm was achieved for the 5 data sets. Figure 7A gives the error color map on the fitted B-spline LA surface. To demonstrate potential use of the LA unfolding method, a lesion map created from the delayed enhancement MRI was used to generate a 2D unfolding color map [14]. This could be used together with MRI-derived LA model guidance to redo ablation procedures as it gives information about previously ablated areas (red regions in figure 7B and 7C).

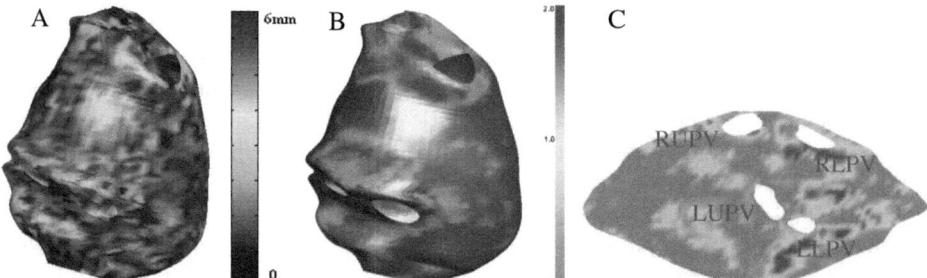

Fig. 7. (A) Color map for surface fitting errors. (B) 3D lesion map created from the delayed enhancement MRI. (Scale for the color bar is the number of standard deviations from the mean of blood pool intensity.) (C) 2D unfolding lesion map.

5   Discussion and Conclusion

This paper describes the implementation of *cardiac unfold* in CRT procedures (LV unfolding) and atrial fibrillation ablation procedures (LA unfolding). The 2D bull's-eye guidance platform for CRT procedures allows simultaneous visualization of the LV and coronary vein morphology, myocardial scar distribution, dyssynchrony information and pacing lead position for the entire LV in real-time. The methodology was validated using 13 data sets from patients that underwent CRT and the accuracy of mapping the pacing lead position to the bull's-eye plot was calculated to be approximately 2 mm, which is well within the requirements of clinical accuracy. The guidance platform was tested on 5 live cases and proved successful to allow navigation for LV lead implantation. Furthermore, the technique of LA surface unfolding was also demonstrated in this paper. The average unfolding error was less than 1 mm in 5 patient data sets. This technique could be useful for navigation since it allows the visualisation of large amounts of complex geometric and functional information in a single 2D representation. It could also be useful if coupled to a robotic catheter system to reduce the degrees of freedom in the control interface.

In conclusion, *cardiac unfold* techniques are promising for augmenting image-based navigation for catheter-based cardiac interventions. Further, validation and testing of these will be required to prove clinical utility.

References

1. Sra, J., Narayan, G., Krum, D., Malloy, A., Cooley, R., Bhatia, A., Dhala, A., Blanck, Z., Nangia, V., Akhtar, M.: Computed tomography-fluoroscopy image integration-guided catheter ablation of atrial fibrillation. Journal of Cardiovascular Electrophysiology 18(4), 409–414 (2007)
2. Rhode, K.S., Hill, D.L.G., Edwards, P.J., Hipwell, J., Rueckert, D., Sanchez-Ortiz, G., Hegde, S., Rahunathan, V., Razavi, R.: Registration and tracking to integrate X-ray and MR images in an XMR facility. IEEE Transactions on Medical Imaging 24(11), 810–815 (2003)
3. Pruemmer, M., Hornegger, J., Lauritsch, G., Wigstrom, L., Girard-Hughes, E., Fahrig, R.: Cardiac C-arm CT: a unified framework for motion estimation and dynamic CT. IEEE Transactions on Medical Imaging 28(11), 1836–1849 (2009)
4. Orlov, M.V., Hoffmeister, P., Chaudhry, G.M., Almasry, I., Gijsbers, G.H., Swack, T., Haffajee, C.I.: Three-dimensional rotational angiography of the left atrium and esophagus–A virtual computed tomography scan in the electrophysiology lab. Heart Rhythm 4(1), 37–43 (2007)
5. Duckett, S.G., Ginks, M.R., et al.: Advanced image fusion to overlay coronary sinus anatomy with real time fluoroscopy to facilitate left ventricular lead implantation in CRT. Pacing Clin. Electrophysiol. 34(2), 226–234 (2010)
6. Ma, Y., Duckett, S., Chinchapatnam, P., Shetty, A., Aldo Rinaldi, C., Schaeffter, T., Rhode, K.S.: Image and Physiological Data Fusion for Guidance and Modelling of Cardiac Resynchronization Therapy Procedures. In: Camara, O., Pop, M., Rhode, K., Sermesant, M., Smith, N., Young, A. (eds.) STACOM 2010. LNCS, vol. 6364, pp. 105–113. Springer, Heidelberg (2010)
7. Manzke, R., Bornstedt, A., et al.: Respiratory motion compensated overlay of surface models from cardiac MR on interventional x-ray fluoroscopy for guidance of cardiac resynchronization therapy procedures. In: SPIE Medical Imaging 2010: Visualization, Image-Guided Procedures, and Modeling, vol. 7625 (2010)
8. Drury, H.A., Van Essen, D.C., et al.: Computerized mappings of the cerebral cortex: a multiresolution flattening method and a surface-based coordinate system. J. Cogn. Neurosci. 8, 1–28 (1996)
9. Termeer, M., Bescós, J.O., Breeuwer, M., Vilanova, A., Gerritsen, F.A., Gröller, M.E., Nagel, E.: Visualization of myocardial perfusion derived from coronary anatomy. IEEE Trans. Vis. Comput. Graph. 14(6), 1595–1602 (2008)
10. Peters, J., Ecabert, O., Meyer, C., Schramm, H., Kneser, R., Groth, A., Weese, J.: Automatic Whole Heart Segmentation in Static Magnetic Resonance Image Volumes. In: Ayache, N., Ourselin, S., Maeder, A. (eds.) MICCAI 2007, Part II. LNCS, vol. 4792, pp. 402–410. Springer, Heidelberg (2007)
11. Ma, Y., Saetzler, K.: A parallelized surface extraction algorithm for large binary image data sets based on adaptive 3-D Delaunay subdivision strategy. IEEE Transactions on Visualization and Computer Graphics 14(1), 160–172 (2008)

12. Karim, R., Mohiaddin, R., Drivas, P., Rueckert, D.: Automatic extraction of the left atrial anatomy from MR for atrial fibrillation ablation. In: Proceedings of IEEE International Symposium on Biomedical Imaging (2009)
13. Ma, Y., King, A., Gogin, N., Gijsbers, G., Rinaldi, C.A., Gill, J., Razavi, R., Rhode, K.: Clinical evaluation of respiratory motion compensation for anatomical roadmap guided cardiac electrophysiology procedures. IEEE Transactions on Biomedical Engineering 59(1), 122–131 (2011)
14. Knowles, B., Caulfield, D., et al.: Three-dimensional visualization of acute radiofrequency ablation lesions using MRI for the simultaneous determination of the patterns of necrosis and edema. IEEE Trans. Biomedical Engineering 57(6), 1467–1475 (2010)

Enabling 3D Ultrasound Procedure Guidance through Enhanced Visualization[*]

Laura J. Brattain[1,2], Nikolay V. Vasilyev[3], and Robert D. Howe[1]

[1] Harvard School of Engineering and Applied Sciences, Cambridge, MA USA 02138
[2] MIT Lincoln Laboratory, 244 Wood St., Lexington, MA USA 02420
[3] Department of Cardiac Surgery, Children's Hospital Boston, Boston, MA USA 02115
{brattain,howe}@seas.harvard.edu,
nikolay.vasilyev@cardio.chboston.org

Abstract. Real-time 3D ultrasound (3DUS) imaging offers improved spatial orientation information relative to 2D ultrasound. However, in order to improve its efficacy in guiding minimally invasive intra-cardiac procedures where real-time visual feedback of an instrument tip location is crucial, 3DUS volume visualization alone is inadequate. This paper presents a set of enhanced visualization functionalities that are able to track the tip of an instrument in slice views at real-time. User study with *in vitro* porcine heart indicates a speedup of over 30% in task completion time.

Keywords: 3D ultrasound, electromagnetic tracking, graphic processing unit, instrument navigation, mosaicing, slice view.

1   Introduction

Real-time 3D ultrasound (3DUS) offers important advantages for guiding diverse medical procedures. Foremost is the ability to visualize complex 3D structures [1]. Studies have shown that real-time 3DUS is more efficient and accurate than 2DUS for basic surgical tasks and can enable more complex procedures [2]. Imaging rates up to 30 volumes per second also enable good visualization of instrument-tissue interactions, far faster than the volumetric imaging alternatives (MR and CT scans). Fluoroscopy provides fast frame rates, but only has a limited number of 2D views, requiring the clinician to mentally combine them to derive 3D structure. Unlike fluoroscopy, 3DUS also allows visualization of the soft tissues, and avoids the use of ionizing radiation. 3DUS is easily integrated into procedures as the small probe can be readily placed at the point of interest. Finally, costs are also far lower, with top-of-the-line 3D ultrasound machines costing far less than comparable fluoroscopy, CT, or MR systems.

Despite these evident advantages, a decade after its commercial introduction, 3DUS is rarely used clinically for procedure guidance. There has been a broad

---

[*] The Harvard University portion of the work is sponsored by US National Institutes of Health under grant NIH R01 HL073647-01. The MIT Lincoln Laboratory portion of the work is sponsored by the Department of the Air Force under Air Force contract #FA8721-05-C-0002. Opinions, interpretations, conclusions and recommendations are those of the author and are not necessarily endorsed by the United States Government.

P. Abolmaesumi et al. (Eds.): IPCAI 2012, LNAI 7330, pp. 115–124, 2012.

spectrum of research in 3DUS guidance, in diverse areas including liver surgery [3] [4], liver ablation [5], kidney imaging [6] and cardiac imaging [7][8][9]. Nonetheless, 2D ultrasound is still the prevailing choice in hospitals [1]. The reasons for this surprising lack of acceptance of 3DUS are diverse. One clear drawback of 3DUS is limited resolution. While voxel sizes are less than one millimeter, noise and distortion typically make it hard to discern features smaller than a few millimeters. In addition, 3DUS images are typically displayed as volume-rendered images. While this is effective for visualizing tissue surfaces surrounded by fluids as in obstetrics and cardiology, volume rendering can accentuate the distortion and noise inherent in 3DUS imaging [10], resulting in irregular surfaces and difficulty in distinguishing instrument artifacts [11][12]. Volume rendering is also problematic for visualizing the internal features of solid organs like liver and kidney, where the entire organ produces textured reflections that fill the imaging volume. Another limitation is the small field of view. Because of the inherent tradeoff in ultrasound imaging between volume size, resolution and frame rate, the volume size is inherently limited.

We hypothesize that enhanced displays can overcome key limitations in current 3DUS guidance, and bring the benefits of 3DUS to a broad range of procedures. One way to address the lack of surface definition and the difficulty in distinguishing instrument from tissue in volume rendered images is to display a cut plane image or "slice" from the 3DUS volume that contains the instrument tip. Because this cross-sectional view shows the point of contact of the instrument with the tissue, as well as adjacent tissue regions, the clinician can determine the specifics of the tool-tissue interaction. Manually selecting planes within the 3DUS volume that contain the instrument tip, however, is highly challenging, particularly as the instrument moves within the volume. The ability to automatically visualize these slice views would greatly enhance the usability of 3DUS.

In addition, research efforts on mosaicing multiple 3DUS volumes to create an extended field of view have been recently reported [13][14]. We further hypothesize that integrating slice views with a mosaiced volume would enable 3DUS for more complex interventions, particularly those requiring navigation across regions larger than a single 3DUS volume.

In this paper, we describe the design of a system for tracking the catheter tip to enable continuous display of exactly the right slices. We report the results of a user study that indicates the potential of such enhanced displays in improving the efficacy of real-time 3DUS guided procedures. In the next section, we present the system design, followed by user study and results. We conclude the paper with a discussion of implications for the design of procedure guidance systems.

2   System Design

2.1   System Configuration

To demonstrate the potential benefits of slice views and mosaicing for procedure guidance, we implemented a prototype visualization system. We used Philips 3DUS scanner iE33 with the X7-2 2D/3D probe, imaging at 8.1cm and 35Hz with a volume size of 112x48x112 voxels (Philips Medical Systems, Andover, MA). An electromagnetic (EM) tracking system (3D Guidance trakStar System, Ascension Technology Corporation, Burlington, VT) tracked the trajectories of the 3DUS probe and the instrument tip. Image processing and rendering (Fig. 1) was done on a GPU

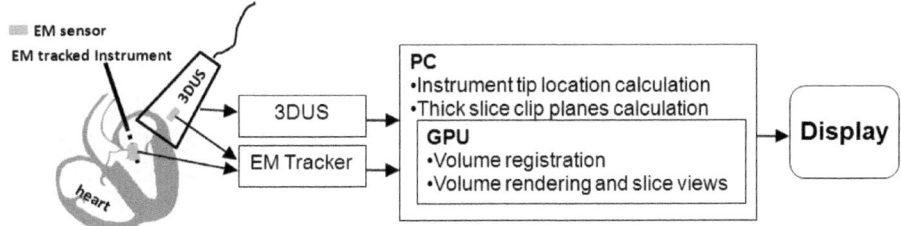

Fig. 1. System Overview

enabled computer (Dell Alienware Aurora, Intel Core i7 processor at 2.67GHz, 6GB RAM, NVIDIA GTX260 graphics card).

2.2   Calculation of the Instrument Tip Inside the 3DUS Volume

The system performs real-time 3DUS volume mosaicing to generate an extended field of view [14]. The instrument tip location can be registered to the mosaiced volume or an input volume. An EM sensor is attached rigidly at the tip of the instrument, with the EM sensor x-axis aligned with the shaft of the instrument. Another EM sensor is attached rigidly to the 3DUS probe. T_{US}^{EM} is the transformation matrix between the 3DUS probe and EM sensor. It is derived through a calibration procedure where we scan a triangle wire frame phantom with known geometric dimensions and perform intensity based registration.

There are three coordinate frames involved in the system: US, EM sensor, and EM transmitter (Fig. 2). Assume P^{US} is the voxel in the ultrasound volume that corresponds to the tip of instrument, $P^{Transmitter}$ is the EM sensor reading from the tip of instrument, and S is the scaling matrix that converts the ultrasound volume from voxel unit to a physical unit. The overall transformation can be established as the multiplication of series homogenous transformation matrices

$$T_{EM}^{Transmitter} \; T_{US}^{EM} \; S P^{US} = P^{Transmitter} \tag{1}$$

The tip location in the ultrasound volume can then be derived as

$$P^{US} = S^{-1} T_{US}^{EM\,-1} T_{EM}^{Transmitter\,-1} P^{Transmitter} \tag{2}$$

EM tracker provides six degree of freedom readings of the sensor location. The orientations of EM sensor's three orthogonal axes ($X_{EM2}, Y_{EM2}, Z_{EM2}$) (Fig. 2) are used to generate the initial orthogonal slice views that contain the instrument tip. Users then have the option to further adjust the orientation and thickness of each of the slice.

2.3   Slice Views

The system tracks the instrument tip position and three orthogonal orientations at real-time. The tip can be displayed in an input volume or within a mosaiced volume using the real-time mosacing techniques we developed [14]. Fig. 3a shows the four input volumes from different point of views that contributed to the mosaiced volume shown in Fig. 3b, where the entire left atrium of a porcine heart can been seen. The tip of instrument is inside the atrium, but blends in with the surrounding tissues. In Fig. 3c, the tip of the instrument is highlighted in green. Cut planes for the slice views can also be visualized as in Fig. 4. Once the desired cut planes are identified, the user can switch to the slice views that shows the tissues highlighted in a different color transfer function as shown in Fig. 5.

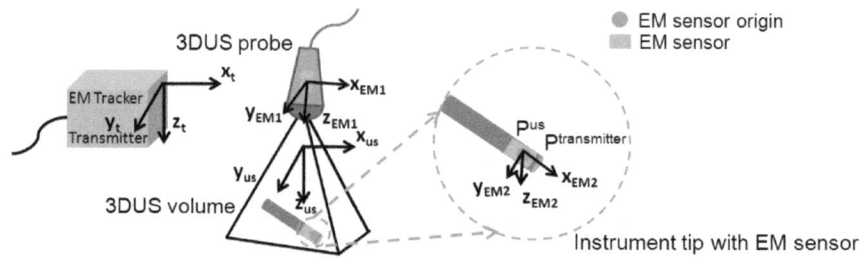

Fig. 2. Coordinate transformations for instrument tip location

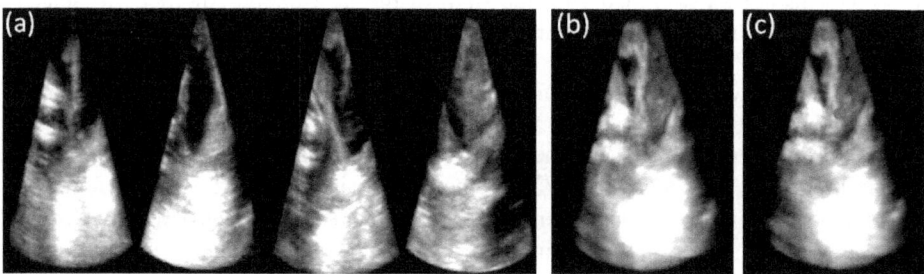

Fig. 3. 3DUS volumes of left atrium. (a) Input volumes. (b) Mosaiced volume with instrument. (c) Mosaiced volume with instrument tip highlighted as a green dot.

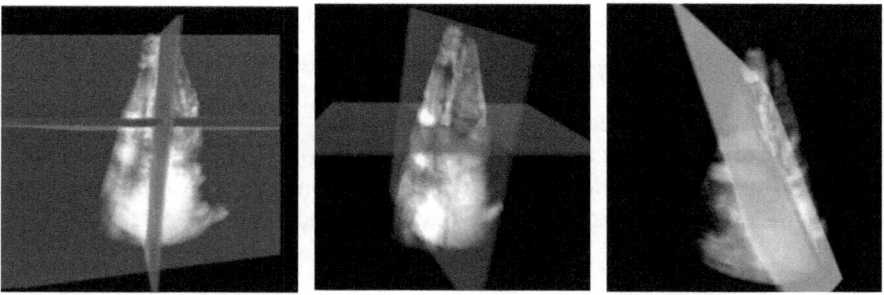

Fig. 4. Orthogonal slice view cut planes through the instrument

3   User Study

We conducted a user study, following a protocol approved by our institutional review board, comparing performance in clinical tasks with and without the enhanced displays. To provide a specific clinical focus, the tasks are taken from intra-cardiac procedures as this specialty shows strong potential for benefiting from 3DUS guidance, however, as discussed below, the proposed display system can apply to a range of other procedures.

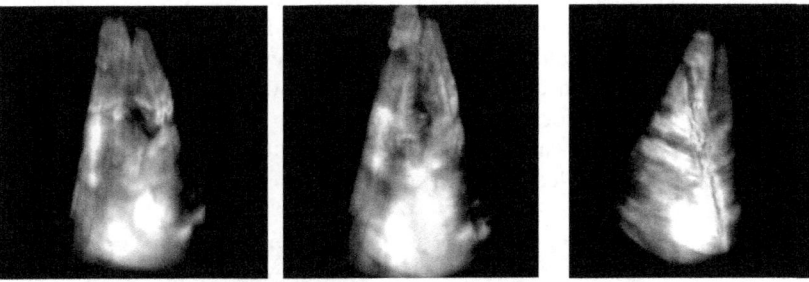

Fig. 5. Orthogonal slice views (in non-gray color map) showing the instrument and its surrounding tissue. The colors correspond to the intensity values.

3.1   Study Design

Five interventional cardiologists with experience in minimally invasive cardiac procedures were recruited for the user study. Their experience in conducting procedures ranged from 3.5 years to 11 years after the beginning of postgraduate training. Each subject performed two instrument navigation tasks in a water tank. Subjects could not directly see the task by eye. There were three 3DUS display conditions: the volume rendered display on the 3DUS machine alone, volume rendered with slice views, and slice views in the mosaiced volume. The order of the tasks and displays for each subject was randomized. In the first two display conditions, subjects moved the probe with one hand to follow the moving instrument and keep it in the 3DUS field of view. With the mosaiced display, there were two options. If the imaging object was static, the user could simply use the EM tracker generated slice views in the mosaic. With moving imaging object, such as a beating heart, the real-time 3DUS volume would be superimposed on the mosaic. In this study, since the image objects were static, subjects did not hold the US probe during the third testing conditions.

Catheter based ablation procedures such as atrial fibrillation (AFib) ablations aim to create linear destructive lesions in the tissue around the pulmonary veins to prevent propagation of an abnormal electrical signal to the rest of the atrial tissue [15]. The first task was to trace the perimeter of the rectangle created by four rubber bands (Fig. 6a) with the tip of a catheter in a water tank. The dimensions of the rectangle were roughly 40mm x 30mm. The goal of this task was to evaluate the effectiveness of the slice views in improving user's ability to maneuver the catheter tip along a predefined path. Rubber bands were chosen because their 3DUS images (Fig. 6b) show significant noise and blurring along the edges, representative of *in vivo* conditions where noise and artifacts are common. The subjects were instructed to hold the catheter roughly 5 cm above its tip, and move the tip along the loop ABCD as outlined in the blue dotted lines in Fig. 6a.

The second task was to trace the mitral annulus of a porcine heart in a water tank using a rigid instrument. An instrument with straight and rigid tip was inserted through a puncture created on the left atrial appendage to access the mitral valve annulus (Fig. 7). In minimally invasive beating heart mitral valve repairs such as mitral annuloplasty, an anchor driver can be inserted through the left atrial appendage to reach the mitral annulus under 3DUS guidance [16]. Although the procedure is promising, instrument tip and tissue often blend together along the atrial wall. This makes it difficult to discern the instrument tip. This task aims to assess the value of slice views and mosaicing for such procedures.

Task completion time was recorded for each subject trial. The instrument tip trajectories were also recorded with EM tracker.

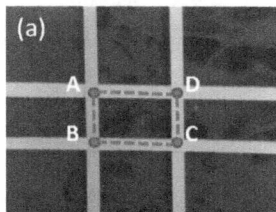 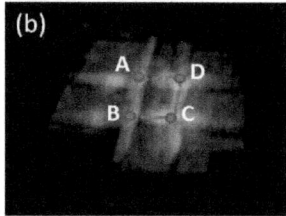

Fig. 6. Navigation task 1. (a) Photograph of the rectangle (40mm x 30 mm) created by four rubber bands. (b) Mosaiced 3DUS image of the four rubber bands containing the rectangle.

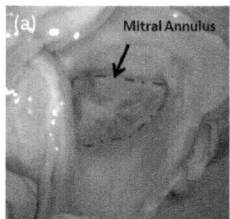 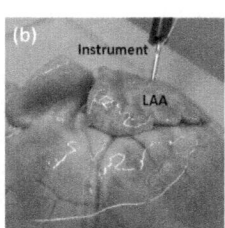 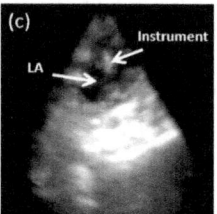

Fig. 7. Navigation task 2. (a) Top down view of the mitral valve and mitral annulus. (b) Instrument inserted through the left atrial appendage (LAA). (c) 3DUS volume rendered showing the left atrium (LA) and part of the instrument.

3.2 Results

Typical trajectories for both tasks are shown in Fig. 8. The completion times from all subject trials were analyzed using Wilcoxon rank sum test (Fig. 9). The criteria for statistical significance was $p \leq 0.05$. The mean deviation of the trajectory (D_{mean}) for task 1 was also calculated by first measuring each line segment AB, BC, CD and

DA (Fig. 6a), and then calculating the mean of the distance from each point on a given trajectory to the corresponding line segment.

In task 1, compared to the completion time under 3DUS volume without slice views, the completion time decreased by 46% with slice views ($p \leq 0.0159$), and D_{mean} decreased by 20%. The completion time decreased by 69% using mosaiced volume with slice views ($p \leq 0.0079$), and D_{mean} decreased by 25%.

In task 2, compared to the completion time under 3DUS volume without slice views, the completion time decreased by 36% with slice views ($p \leq 0.0317$). The completion time decreased by 46% using mosaiced volume with slice views ($p \leq 0.0159$). In both tasks, the variability of the results (standard error) also decreased with enhanced displays. This suggests that with slice and mosaic displays, the surgical task is less dependent on each user's individual echocardiography skills and experience.

Subjects reported that the three orthogonal views were intuitive. All subjects stated that mosaiced volumes combined with slice views have great potential for 3DUS guided interventions.

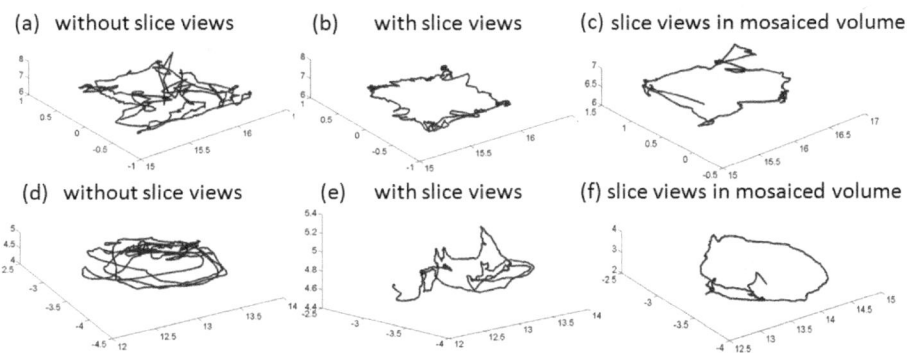

Fig. 8. Typical instrument tip trajectory. (a) - (c) Trajectory of tracing the rectangle rubber bands. (d) - (f) Trajectory of tracing the mitral annulus.

4   Discussion

In this paper, we aim to address the following three key issues in current 3DUS guidance: (1) Volume rendering alone is not adequate to visualize tool-tissue interaction; (2) Slice view avoids problem with volume rendering, but is difficult to align manually; (3) 3DUS has a small field of view and is difficult to navigate. Our prototype system and user study demonstrate that improved visualization techniques could mitigate key limitations in 3DUS. A mosaiced volume overcomes 3DUS limited field of view and can be used for broad navigation. Computer assisted instrument tip tracking in slice views facilitates real-time instrument navigation and visual feedback.

The slice view features developed are still in the research stage. Further development is needed to ultimately improve the end user's experience. The tasks used here are simpler than clinical catheter based procedures and 3DUS imaging in a water tank has better quality than *in vivo* situations. Thus, we expect even better user improvement with slice views and mosaicing in *in vivo* and clinical procedures.

A number of image-guidance systems share features with the approach presented here. For example, 3DSlicer [17], was originally applied to neurosurgery, where tracked instrument positions are superimposed on static preoperative brain images. These systems necessarily used slice views. Similarly, ultrasound visualization tools such as Stradwin and Stradx [18] work with prerecorded data. The system proposed here, however, uses real time volumetric data, which presents significant challenges for real-time registration, mosaicing, and tracking.

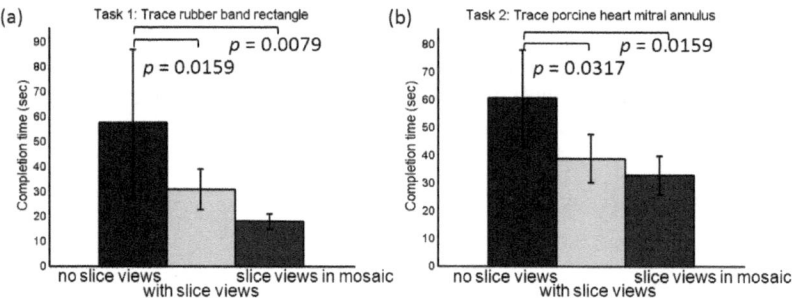

Fig. 9. Task completion times. (a) Task 1 – trace rubber band rectangle. (b) Task 2 – Trace porcine heart mitral annulus.

4.1   System Extensions

Novotny *et al.* developed a GPU based real-time instrument detection algorithm that uses a generalized Radon transform [19]. Any such image-based tracking approach can be advantageously integrated with the current EM tracker based slice views. The EM sensor provides the initial estimate of the tip location, which reduces the image search space hence further speed up the algorithm.

Accuracy of the volume mosaicing could also be further improved using image based methods. Schneider *et al.* developed a real-time feature-based 3DUS registration framework on GPU [20]. Grau *et al.* reported a structure orientation and phase based algorithm to register apical and parasternal 3DUS datasets of the heart [21]. EM based volume registration can be used as an initial estimate for either of these two algorithms.

4.2   Application to Beating Heart Procedures

The slice views presented here can be integrated with an ECG gated mosaicing system for beating heart intra-cardiac procedures [14]. ECG gating captures the heart motion in a complete cardiac cycle.

Currently in a typical catheter based AFib ablation procedure, a 3D electrophysiological model resembling the shape of the atria is generated by recording the locations of the ablation catheter's tip in space. The point clouds are then registered to a CT or MRI based pre-operative anatomic model (e.g. CARTO, Biosense Webster, Diamond Bar, CA). However, this mapping and model creation can be a tedious process and fluoroscopy is routinely used. An ECG gated 3DUS mosaicing system combined with enhanced user display such as slice views could shorten the procedure time, reduce human exposure to fluoroscopy, and provide improved visualization on tool-tissue interaction.

5   Conclusion

In this paper, we presented a set of enhanced display modalities for real-time 3DUS visualization. The system integrates EM tracking systems and GPU implementation for real-time instrument tip cut plane tracking to mitigate the 3DUS distortions inherent in conventional volume rendering. Our user study and participants' feedback demonstrate the potential of such enhanced visualization in instrument navigation and procedure execution with 3DUS guidance.

References

1. Prager, R.W., Ijaz, U.Z., Gee, A.H., Treece, G.M.: Three-dimensional ultrasound imaging. Proc. IMechE Part H: J. Engineering in Medicine 224, 193 (2010)
2. Cannon, J.W., Stoll, J.A., Salgo, I.S., Knowles, H.B., Howe, R.D., Dupont, P.E., Marx, G.R., del Nido, P.J.: Real-time three dimensional ultrasound for guiding surgical tasks. Computer Aided Surgery 8(2), 82–90 (2003)
3. Nakamoto, M., Sato, Y., Miyamoto, M., Nakamjima, Y., Konishi, K., Shimada, M., Hashizume, M., Tamura, S.: 3D Ultrasound System Using a Magneto-optic Hybrid Tracker for Augmented Reality Visualization in Laparoscopic Liver Surgery. In: Dohi, T., Kikinis, R. (eds.) MICCAI 2002, Part II. LNCS, vol. 2489, pp. 148–155. Springer, Heidelberg (2002)
4. Lange, T., Eulenstein, S., Hünerbein, M., Lamecker, H., Schlag, P.-M.: Augmenting Intraoperative 3D Ultrasound with Preoperative Models for Navigation in Liver Surgery. In: Barillot, C., Haynor, D.R., Hellier, P. (eds.) MICCAI 2004, Part II. LNCS, vol. 3217, pp. 534–541. Springer, Heidelberg (2004)
5. Boctor, E.M., Fichtinger, G., Taylor, R.H., Choti, M.A.: Tracked 3D ultrasound in radiofrequency liver ablation. In: Walker, W.F., Insana, M.F. (eds.) Proceedings of the SPIE Ultrasonic Imaging and Signal Processing, Medical Imaging 2003, vol. 5035, pp. 174–182. SPIE, Bellingham (2003)
6. Leroy, A., Mozer, P., Payan, Y., Troccaz, J.: Rigid Registration of Freehand 3D Ultrasound and CT-Scan Kidney Images. In: Barillot, C., Haynor, D.R., Hellier, P. (eds.) MICCAI 2004, Part I. LNCS, vol. 3216, pp. 837–844. Springer, Heidelberg (2004)
7. Huang, X., Hill, N.A., Ren, J., Guiraudon, G., Boughner, D., Peters, T.M.: Dynamic 3D Ultrasound and MR Image Registration of the Beating Heart. In: Duncan, J.S., Gerig, G. (eds.) MICCAI 2005, Part II. LNCS, vol. 3750, pp. 171–178. Springer, Heidelberg (2005)
8. Mor-Avi, V., Sugeng, L., Lang, R.M.: Three dimensional adult echocardiography: where the hidden dimension helps. Current Cardiol. Rep. 10(3), 218–225 (2008)

9. Yagel, S., Cohen, S.M., Shapiro, I., Valsky, D.V.: 3D and 4D ultrasound in fetal cardiac scanning: a new look at the fetal heart. Ultrasound Obstet. Gynecol. 29, 81–95 (2007)
10. Huang, J., Triedman, J.K., Vasilyev, N.V., Suematsu, Y., Cleveland, R.O., Dupont, P.E.: Imaging artifacts of medical instruments in ultrasound-guided interventions. J. Ultrasound Med. 26(10), 1303–1322 (2007)
11. Novotny, P.M., Jacobsen, S.K., Vasilyev, N.V., Kettler, D.T., Salgo, I.S., Dupont, P.E., Del Nido, P.J., Howe, R.D.: 3D ultrasound in robotic surgery: performance evaluation with stereo displays. Int. J. Med. Robotics Comput. Assist. Surg. 2, 279–285 (2006)
12. Mung, J., Vignon, F., Jain, A.: A non-disruptive technology for robust 3D tool tracking for ultrasound-guided interventions. Med. Image Comput. Comput. Assist. Interv. 14(Pt 1), 153–160 (2011)
13. King, A.P., Ma, Y.L., Yao, C., Jansen, C., Razavi, R., Rhode, K.S., Penney, G.P.: Image-to-physical registration for image-guided interventions using 3-D ultrasound and an ultrasound imaging model. Information Processing in Medical Imaging 21, 188–201 (2009)
14. Brattain, L.J., Howe, R.D.: Real-Time 4D Ultrasound Mosaicing and Visualization. In: Fichtinger, G., Martel, A., Peters, T. (eds.) MICCAI 2011, Part I. LNCS, vol. 6891, pp. 105–112. Springer, Heidelberg (2011)
15. Hocini, M., Jaïs, P., Sanders, P., Takahashi, Y., Rotter, M., Rostock, T., Hsu, L.F., Sacher, F., Reuter, S., Clémenty, J., Haïssaguerre, M.: Techniques, evaluation, and consequences of linear block at the left atrial roof in paroxysmal atrial fibrillation: a prospective randomized study. Circulation 112, 3688–3696 (2005)
16. Yuen, S.G., Kesner, S.B., Vasilyev, N.V., Del Nido, P.J., Robert, D., Howe, R.D.: 3D Ultrasound-Guided Motion Compensation System for Beating Heart Mitral Valve Repair. Med. Image Comput. Comput. Assist. Interv. 11(Pt 1), 711–719 (2008)
17. 3D Slicer, http://www.slicer.org/
18. Free software from the medical imaging group, http://mi.eng.cam.ac.uk/~rwp/Software.html
19. Novotny, P.M., Stoll, J.A., Vasilyev, N.V., Del Nido, P.J., Dupont, P.E., Zickler, T.E., Howe, R.D.: GPU based real-time instrument tracking with three-dimensional ultrasound. Medical Image Analysis 11, 458–464 (2007)
20. Schneider, R.J., Perrin, D.P., Vasilyev, N.V., Marx, G.R., Del Nido, P.J., Howe, R.D.: Real-time image-based rigid registration of three-dimensional ultrasound. Medical Image Analysis 16(2), 402–414 (2012); ISSN 1361-8415, doi:10.1016/j.media.2011.10.004
21. Grau, V., Becher, H., Noble, J.A.: Registration of Multiview Real-time 3-D Echocardiographic Sequences. IEEE Trans. on Medical Imaging 26(9) (September 2007)

Fast and Robust Registration Based on Gradient Orientations: Case Study Matching Intra-operative Ultrasound to Pre-operative MRI in Neurosurgery

Dante De Nigris[1], D. Louis Collins[2], and Tal Arbel[1]

[1] McGill University, Centre for Intelligent Machines
{dante,tal}@cim.mcgill.ca
[2] Montreal Neurological Institute, McGill University, Montreal, Canada
louis.collins@mcgill.ca

Abstract. We present a novel approach for the rigid registration of pre-operative magnetic resonance to intra-operative ultrasound in the context of image-guided neurosurgery. Our framework proposes the maximization of gradient orientation alignment in locations with minimal uncertainty of the orientation estimates, permitting fast and robust performance. We evaluated our method on 14 clinical neurosurgical cases of patients with brain tumors, including low-grade and high-grade gliomas. We demonstrate processing times as small as 7 seconds and improved performance with relation to competing intensity-based methods.

Keywords: Image Registration, Neurosurgery, Ultrasound.

1 Introduction

In image-guided neurosurgery (IGNS), brain deformations during open craniotomies, commonly known as brain shifts, reduce the accuracy of pre-operative images used for guidance. Using intra-operative magnetic resonance imaging (MRI) to overcome this problem presents several disadvantages including a prohibitive cost, and cumbersome and intrusive changes to the operating theater and standard procedures. Intra-operative ultrasound (iUS) has been proposed in recent years as a practical, less invasive and less expensive alternative to estimate the deformations [2]. However, US images typically show reduced image quality, fewer anatomical details and are generally harder to interpret. In order to benefit from both the imaging detail and resolution of MRI and the practical advantages of US, a number of groups have proposed different methods to register the pre-operative MRI volume to an iUS volume [2,8,11,12,16]. The estimated deformation can then be used to provide the surgeon with an updated MRI volume suitable for guidance. For this strategy to be adopted in clinical practice, the registration results are required to be both accurate and robust to patient variability. In addition, the technique should have relatively short processing times so as to minimize the overhead in the surgical procedure.

P. Abolmaesumi et al. (Eds.): IPCAI 2012, LNAI 7330, pp. 125–134, 2012.

The alignment of MRI to iUS images is particularly challenging due to the widely different nature and quality of the modalities involved. In MRI, each voxel's intensity is to a large extent a direct function of the tissue type found within the voxel's volume. Alternatively, US image intensities are actually a function of the probe's direction (i.e. direction of the sound wave) and the presence of an acoustic impedance transition. Fig. 1 shows an MRI volume and a corresponding iUS volume of a case involving a brain tumor. Notice the challenge in relating one image to another. The MRI volume permits the accurate and precise identification of multiple tissue types and anatomical structures (e.g. brain tumor, white matter, gray matter and bone tissue). On the other hand, iUS is mostly limited to exposing tumor tissue with an associated uncertainty regarding its boundary, along with a few coarsely depicted structure boundaries.

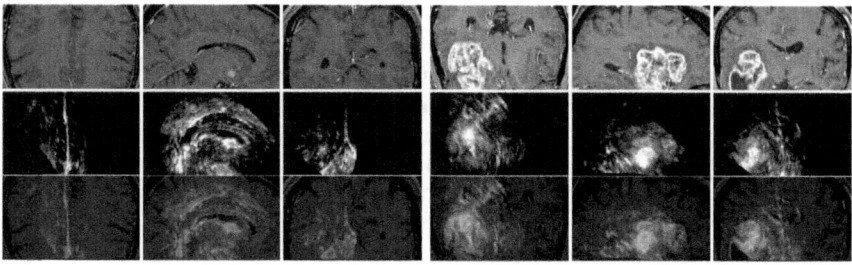

Fig. 1. Image slices from a pre-operative MRI volume and a corresponding iUS volume in a brain tumor resection surgery. The top row shows the MRI. The middle row shows the iUS. The third row shows the iUS with a heat color mapping overlayed onto the MRI at their initial, unregistered positions. Notice the misalignment between key structures such as along the longitudinal fissure.

In order to perform registration in this context, previous techniques have mostly relied on intensity-based similarity metrics such as mutual information (MI), normalized cross correlation (NCC) and normalized mutual information (NMI). However, due to the challenges brought forward by US, most authors also include a pre-processing stage which transforms the original images to feature images with a potentially increased likelihood of having a correspondence throughout the *full* spatial domain. For example, some approaches maximize the correspondence between the gradient magnitude of both images [3]. Similarly, in [14], the authors employ a similarity metric based on an inferred mapping from the MRI voxel intensity and gradient magnitude to the US voxel intensity, while in [16], the authors choose to maximize the MI of the local phase.

Unfortunately, such local features are ultimately tightly coupled to the pixel intensity response of each modality, and thus also tend to exhibit a variable response with relation to corresponding anatomical structures in US. This can be observed in Fig. 1, where image intensities and corresponding gradient magnitudes of the longitudinal fissure and lateral ventricles depicted in the US images vary greatly throughout the spatial domain, dropping to null values in some regions. As a result, traditional registration techniques that build *global* models for the two modalities, based on the assumption of homogeneous image features, will necessarily see a degradation of performance in this context.

Other approaches rely on more elaborate pre-processing stages or the simulation of US. In [2,12], the authors construct a pseudo-US from the MRI which is then registered to the iUS by maximization of the cross correlation. The pseudo-US is obtained by hard-mapping automatically segmented tissue types from the MRI to intensity values that have been defined *a priori* and then blurring the obtained image. In [11], the authors choose to non-linearly filter the US and restrict its domain by manually defining a region of interest around the tumor. The resulting image is then registered by maximizing the MI value. Similarly, in [8], the authors apply a median filter to the MRI, blur the US with a Gaussian kernel, restrict the domain with a mask of high-intensity regions in the US and then maximize the NMI value. In [15], the authors address the registration of US to CT with the use of a simulated US obtained from the CT. Unfortunately, the approach relies on a hard-mapping of the CT intensity to the tissue's echogeneity, and a comparable strategy in the context of IGNS can easily break down. In particular, the dependence on fixed mappings between intensities represents a sensitivity to variations of the image formation model. This is a critical concern in IGNS where each case has unique US imaging parameters (e.g. probe direction and focal point depth) related to the size and location of the tumor. Each patient can also have a unique pathology, leading to unpredictable US to MRI intensity characteristics, particularly around the pathology where the accuracy is required the most. These methods have demonstrated improved performance, yet typically require fine-tuning for each context and don't generalize well.

In this paper, we propose a new MRI to US registration framework, with the goal of providing substantially improved robustness and computational performance in the context of IGNS. Registration is based on gradient orientation alignment, in order to reduce the effect of the non-homogeneous intensity response found in US. However, orientation estimates can be noisy in this context and using the full set of orientations would lead to undue computational cost and risk of errors. In order to address such limitations, our technique first selects locations whose gradient orientations have high certainty (i.e. minimal noise) and likely correspond to structures of interest. Once such locations have been identified, we maximize their alignment with corresponding orientations.

Experimental findings show that our approach brings forward gains in computational performance and registration accuracy. In particular, we can achieve a robust performance, in the sense that all 14 cases have a resulting mean distance between corresponding points that is larger than the smallest possible mean distance (under a rigid transformation) by no more than 1 mm. Furthermore, such performance is achieved with a highly reduced subset of voxels (e.g. 2% of the image), leading to an average processing time of 10 seconds. This achievement should permit the strategy to be embedded in the clinical IGNS system.

2   Methodology

The proposed registration method is composed of a local similarity measure based on gradient orientation alignment (GOA), which evaluates the similarity between the gradient of the fixed image, ∇I_F, and moving image, ∇I_M, as,

$$GOA(\nabla I_F, \nabla I_M) = \cos{(\Delta\theta)}^2 \qquad (1)$$

where $\Delta\theta$ is the inner angle between ∇I_F and ∇I_M. Similar metrics can be found in previous work [5,6,9].

Ideally, we should make sole use of gradient orientations that actually reflect the direction of anatomical boundaries and disregard all gradient orientations brought forward by image artifacts or noise. An intuitive choice for an indicator of the reliability of a gradient orientation is the image gradient magnitude, since locations with high gradient magnitude tend to visually correspond to anatomical boundaries of interest. We can also demonstrate that under the assumption of i.i.d. additive Gaussian noise on voxel intensities, the gradient magnitude actually corresponds inversely to the variance of the corresponding gradient orientation.[1] Thus, we use the gradient magnitude as an indicator of the certainty of each gradient orientation, and restrict the evaluation of the similarity metric to locations with high gradient magnitudes.

We also simplify the computation of the gradient of the transformed moving image by simply mapping the gradients from the original (i.e. not transformed) moving image. In other words, instead of re-computing image gradients at each evaluated transformation by resampling voxel intensities and recomputing derivatives, we compute image gradients only once. The linear mapping of image gradients can be easily found by expanding the expression for the image derivative of a transformed moving image. Consider a D-dimensional moving image, I_M, whose coordinate space is *inversely* mapped by a continuous transformation function, $\mathbf{T}$, to the fixed image coordinate space. In other words, a location, $\mathbf{x} = (x_1, \ldots, x_D)$, in the fixed image coordinate space corresponds to location $\mathbf{T}(\mathbf{x}) = (T_1, \ldots, T_D)$ in the coordinate space of the original moving image. The derivative of the moving image with respect to a particular dimension, x_j, of the fixed image coordinate space, is expressed as,

$$\left.\frac{\partial I_m}{\partial x_j}\right|_{\mathbf{T}(\mathbf{x})} = \sum_i^D \left.\frac{\partial I_m}{\partial T_i}\right|_{\mathbf{T}(\mathbf{x})} \cdot \left.\frac{\partial T_i}{\partial x_j}\right|_{\mathbf{x}} \qquad (2)$$

where the term $\frac{\partial T_i}{\partial x_j}$ corresponds to the (i,j)-th component of the spatial Jacobian matrix of the transformation function.

$$J_{\mathbf{T}} = \begin{bmatrix} \dfrac{\partial T_1}{\partial x_1} & \cdots & \dfrac{\partial T_1}{\partial x_D} \\ \vdots & \ddots & \vdots \\ \dfrac{\partial T_D}{\partial x_1} & \cdots & \dfrac{\partial T_D}{\partial x_D} \end{bmatrix}. \qquad (3)$$

---

[1] Proof for this has been omitted due to restrictions in space.

Re-arranging the terms we obtain the expression for the transformed image gradient,

$$\nabla_{\mathbf{x}} I_m\big(\mathbf{T}(\mathbf{x})\big) = J_{\mathbf{T}}^T(\mathbf{x}) \cdot \nabla_{\mathbf{T}} I_m\big(\mathbf{T}(\mathbf{x})\big) \tag{4}$$

where $\nabla_{\mathbf{T}} I_m(\mathbf{x}) = \left(\frac{\partial I_m(\mathbf{T}(\mathbf{x}))}{\partial T_1}, \ldots, \frac{\partial I_m(\mathbf{T}(\mathbf{x}))}{\partial T_D} \right)$ is the gradient of the original moving image. The gradient of the transformed moving image is therefore evaluated as the product of the transpose of the spatial Jacobian matrix and the gradient of the original (undeformed) moving image.

3   Clinical Data

Registration was performed on 14 clinical cases of patients involving low and high-grade gliomas at various depths and locations in the brain which form part of a soon-to-be publicly available dataset [1]. Each case includes: a pre-operative MRI volume, a set of 2D iUS images, a reconstructed 3D iUS volume, and a set of manually identified corresponding landmarks. The study was approved by the local Institutional Research Ethics Board and written informed consent was obtained from each subject prior to study initiation.

All cases involve the registration of a pre-operative MRI volume to a iUS volume where the initial location corresponds to a preliminary registration involving the manual identification of homologous landmarks on the skin and the MRI volume. Two-dimensional US images were acquired with an HDI 5000 machine on the dura prior to resection, where the probe was tracked with reflective spheres rigidly fixed to a tracker and using a Polaris infrared optical system. The 2D images are captured through a Pinnacle PCTV frame-grabbing card, with each acquisition sweep containing between 200 and 600 frames. A 3D iUS volume was then reconstructed using a pixel-based method, mapping US pixels to a 3D grid with a voxel spacing of 1.0×1.0×1.0 mm. The reconstruction of the 3D US volume currently represents a significant delay with an average processing time of 90 seconds, to a large extent due to lack of code optimization. However, we note that real-time 3D US reconstruction was recently demonstrated in [4].

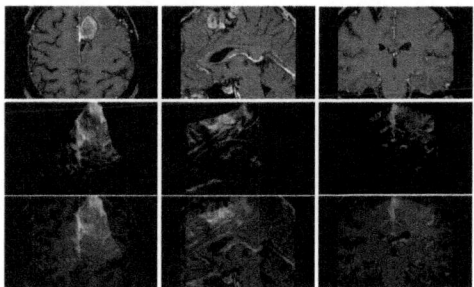

Fig. 2. Case 10 after registration with proposed approach

Registration performance is measured as the mean distance between anatomically corresponding points independently identified by two or three experts, as is standard clinical practice. The total number of landmarks per case ranges between 19 and 40. It is important to note that given both the uncertainty of accurately identifying anatomical locations in the US volume as well as the potential presence of non-rigid components in the transformation, the minimal mean distance between points under a rigid transformation is generally not zero and varies from case to case. For reference purposes, we also demonstrate the minimal mean distance for each case in the experiments sections, which is effectively the lower bound on the performance metric under a rigid transformation.

4   Experiments

We evaluated our approach with two different configurations. Preliminary empirical evaluations have shown that the performance of the method is not particularly sensitive to the percentage of locations selected, yielding similar results when choosing at least the top 10% locations (with highest gradient magnitude). Smaller selection rates (e.g. top 1%) tend to identify highly clustered locations that correspond to one particular boundary, thereby compromising registration robustness. However, we do demonstrate that we can improve computational efficiency without sacrificing robustness by randomly choosing a reduced subset of locations within a sampling mask. For the purpose of brevity, we will only demonstrate registration results corresponding to selecting the top 20% locations in the image or a reduced random subset of location within such sampling mask.

The first configuration, (GOA Full), involves maximizing the mean gradient orientation alignment of the full sampling mask defined by 20% of the voxels in the volume with highest gradient magnitude. The optimization of the metric is performed with a covariance matrix adaptation evolution strategy (CAE)[7], a non-gradient based optimization strategy. We have defined the stopping criterion to be a change in the metric value smaller than 10^{-6}.

The second configuration, (GOA Subset), is meant to yield further reduced processing times but with potentially inferior accuracy. In particular, instead of using all the voxels in the top 20% sampling mask, we randomly select a subset of 8000 voxels within the mask, which constitute around 2% of the total number of US voxels in the 3D volume. Furthermore, we also change the stopping criterion of the optimization to be a change in the metric value smaller than 10^{-3}.

For comparison purposes, we also demonstrate the performance of conventional registration techniques. Recently proposed US specific registration techniques [15,16] were not evaluated due to implementation challenges (e.g. source code not available, parameter tuning). First, we evaluate intensity-based approaches such as the maximization of normalized cross correlation (NCC), mutual information (MI), and normalized mutual information (NMI). In order to decouple the choice of intensity based similarity metric from optimization techniques, we demonstrate the registration performance of each metric with the same non-gradient based optimization strategy we employ in our method, as well as a gradient-descent (GD) strategy with an adaptive gain.

Table 1. Rigid registration results with proposed method evaluated in 14 clinical cases. Performance is evaluated as the mean distance between manually identified corresponding anatomical points. The first configuration, GOA FULL, involves a sampling mask defined by the top 20% voxels with highest gradient magnitude in the US. The second configuration, GOA SUBSET, restricts the evaluation of the metric to a random subset of 8000 voxels found within the top 20% sampling mask. Also shown are the initial and minimal mean distance. The minimal mean distance is the smallest possible value for the mean distance between points under a rigid transformation.

Case	Initial	Minimal	GOA Full		GOA Subset	
	Distance	Distance	Distance	Time	Distance	Time
1	4.89	3.93	4.89	53 s	4.86	12 s
2	6.45	1.60	1.79	50 s	1.78	9 s
3	9.38	2.48	2.73	76 s	2.65	16 s
4	3.93	1.62	1.68	37 s	1.72	7 s
5	2.63	1.91	2.12	36 s	2.13	9 s
6	2.30	1.50	1.81	48 s	1.71	9 s
7	3.04	2.06	2.51	48 s	2.64	14 s
8	3.59	2.37	2.63	56 s	2.65	10 s
9	5.09	2.30	2.70	40 s	2.79	7 s
10	2.97	1.75	1.95	73 s	1.94	9 s
11	1.52	1.33	1.56	52 s	1.82	9 s
12	3.70	2.36	2.64	41 s	2.47	8 s
13	5.15	3.20	3.47	43 s	3.42	12 s
14	3.77	2.33	2.94	62 s	2.92	9 s
Average	4.17	2.20	2.53	51 s	2.54	10 s
Median	3.74	2.18	2.57	49 s	2.55	9 s

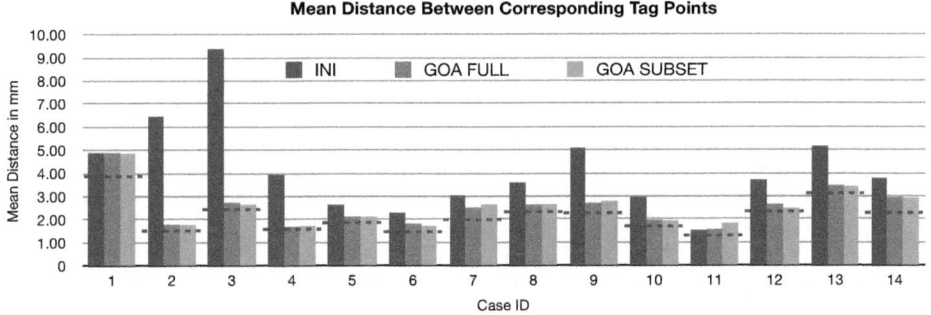

Fig. 3. Rigid registration results with proposed method evaluated with 14 clinical cases. The x-axis corresponds to the clinical case, while the y-axis corresponds to the mean distance between manually identified corresponding anatomical points. Also shown are the initial mean distance, (INI), in blue, as well as the minimal mean distance (MIN) possible under a rigid transformation, shown as a red dashed line.

We also evaluate registration performance when the gradient magnitude images are used as input images instead of the original volumes and the same intensity-based similarity metrics are employed. Finally, we implement a technique based on the work found in [8]. This approach involves a more sophisticated pre-processing stage in which the MRI volume is processed with a median filter and the US volume is Gaussian blurred to reduce the effect of speckle. Next, a sampling mask for the US volume is obtained by first identifying the voxels with intensity values above the Otsu threshold[13], and consequently dilating the obtained mask. The resulting images are then registered by maximization of NMI. We note that all registration methods were evaluated with *Elastix* [10] based tools on a Linux machine with an Intel Core2 Quad Processor Q6700.

Table 2. Statistical summary of rigid registration results with all evaluated techniques. The first column identifies the method used which is characterized by a similarity metric (e.g. Mutual Information (MI), Normalized Cross Correlation (NCC), Normalized Mutual Information (NMI) and Gradient Orientation Alignment (GOA)), input images (e.g. Original Images (ORI), Gradient Magnitude Images (GM) and Median Filtered MRI in conjunction with a Gaussian blurred US (PRE)) and optimization strategy (e.g. Covariance-Matrix-Adaptation-Evolution-Strategy (CAE) and a Gradient Descent (GD) optimizer with adaptive gain). The first two columns of registration results show the average and median value of the mean distance between manually identified corresponding points. Also shown are the average and median value of the mean distance minus the minimal mean distance and the number of cases in which the mean distance is larger than the minimal mean distance by no more than 1 or 2 mm.

Method	Mean		Mean - Minimal		Nbr of Successes	
	Average	Median	Average	Median	<1mm	<2mm
MI+ORI+CAE	22.62	9.20	20.42	7.51	3	3
NMI+ORI+CAE	21.58	8.63	19.39	6.89	3	4
NCC+ORI+CAE	70.58	76.30	68.38	74.11	0	0
MI+ORI+GD	11.83	6.84	9.64	4.44	3	5
NMI+ORI+GD	11.68	6.88	9.64	4.44	3	5
NCC+ORI+GD	37.83	29.73	35.63	28.21	0	0
MI+GM+CAE	3.00	2.90	0.81	0.64	9	12
NMI+GM+CAE	3.01	2.78	0.82	0.59	10	12
NCC+GM+CAE	6.59	3.09	4.39	0.79	8	11
MI+GM+GD	2.90	2.67	0.71	0.61	11	14
NMI+GM+GD	2.87	2.66	0.67	0.60	12	13
NCC+GM+GD	3.77	2.91	1.57	0.69	9	12
NMI+PRE+CAE	13.47	9.22	11.28	6.83	0	1
NMI+PRE+GD	10.78	8.67	8.59	5.83	0	0
GOA+FULL	**2.53**	**2.57**	**0.33**	**0.27**	**14**	**14**
GOA+SUBSET	**2.54**	**2.55**	**0.34**	**0.22**	**14**	**14**

Table 1 lists the registration results for all 14 cases of our proposed approach with both configurations. The same set of results is also illustrated in Fig. 3. Notice that both configurations consistently reduce the mean distance from its initial point and that the resulting mean distance is actually quite close to the minimal mean distance under a rigid transformation. The processing times of the first configuration, (GOA Full), range from 36 to 76 seconds, comparable to the processing time of intensity-based methods. However, we see that by reducing the number of evaluated voxels and relaxing the stopping criterion in the second configuration, (GOA Subset), we obtain a similar registration performance with much shorter processing times that range from 7 to 14 seconds.

Table 2 summarizes the registration performance of all evaluated methods. In particular, we demonstrate the average and median value of two performance metrics: the mean distance between manually identified points, and the difference between the mean distance and the minimal mean distance. We also show the number of cases with successful registrations, where we define success as the case when the mean distance between points is larger than the minimal mean distance by no more than 1 or 2 mm. Notice that common intensity-based similarity metrics, like MI, NCC, and NMI, generally have very poor performance with both optimization strategies. However, if we employ a gradient magnitude image with the same similarity metrics, we begin to obtain more satisfactory results. In particular, maximizing NMI between the gradient magnitude images with a gradient-descent strategy, manages to register 12 of the 14 cases with a mean distance less than 1mm larger than the minimal mean distance. Both configurations of our proposed approach manage to resolve all cases with a mean distance less than 1 mm larger than the minimal mean distance. Furthermore, the median difference between the obtained mean distance and minimal mean distance is of 0.27 mm for the first configuration, (GOA Full) and 0.22 mm for the second, (GOA Subset).

5   Conclusion

In this paper, we have presented a new and robust approach for the rigid registration of pre-operative MRI volumes to iUS volumes which provides fast performance. All 14 clinical cases evaluated were successfully registered with a median difference between the mean distance after registration and the minimal distance (i.e. lower bound) of 0.22 mm. Our method is also computationally efficient since it does not require additional pre-processing stages and can resolve the transformation with the evaluation of a very small percentage of locations (e.g. 2%) with registration times as low as 7 seconds.

References

1. Anonymous: Online database of clinical MR and ultrasound images of brain tumours. Submitted to Medical Physics (October 2011)
2. Arbel, T., Morandi, X., Comeau, R.M., Collins, D.L.: Automatic Non-linear MRI-Ultrasound Registration for the Correction of Intra-operative Brain Deformations. In: Niessen, W.J., Viergever, M.A. (eds.) MICCAI 2001. LNCS, vol. 2208, pp. 913–922. Springer, Heidelberg (2001)

3. Brooks, R., Collins, D.L., Morandi, X., Arbel, T.: Deformable Ultrasound Registration without Reconstruction. In: Metaxas, D., Axel, L., Fichtinger, G., Székely, G. (eds.) MICCAI 2008, Part II. LNCS, vol. 5242, pp. 1023–1031. Springer, Heidelberg (2008)

4. Dai, Y., Tian, J., Dong, D., Yan, G., Zheng, H.: Real-time visualized freehand 3d ultrasound reconstruction based on gpu. IEEE Transactions on Information Technology in Biomedicine 14(6), 1338–1345 (2010)

5. De Nigris, D., Mercier, L., Del Maestro, R., Louis Collins, D., Arbel, T.: Hierarchical Multimodal Image Registration Based on Adaptive Local Mutual Information. In: Jiang, T., Navab, N., Pluim, J.P.W., Viergever, M.A. (eds.) MICCAI 2010, Part II. LNCS, vol. 6362, pp. 643–651. Springer, Heidelberg (2010)

6. Haber, E., Modersitzki, J.: Beyond mutual information: A simple and robust alternative. In: Meinzer, H.P., Handels, H., Horsch, A., Tolxdorff, T. (eds.) Bildverarbeitung für die Medizin 2005. Informatik aktuell. Springer (2005)

7. Hansen, N., Ostermeier, A.: Completely derandomized self-adaptation in evolution strategies. Evol. Comput. 9, 159–195 (2001)

8. Ji, S., Wu, Z., Hartov, A., Roberts, D.W., Paulsen, K.D.: Mutual-information-based image to patient re-registration using intraoperative ultrasound in image-guided neurosurgery. Medical Physics 35(10), 4612–4624 (2008)

9. Karaçali, B.: Information theoretic deformable registration using local image information. IJCV 72, 219–237 (2007)

10. Klein, S., Staring, M., Murphy, K., Viergever, M., Pluim, J.: elastix: a toolbox for intensity-based medical image registration. IEEE Transactions on Medical Imaging 29(1), 196–205 (2010)

11. Letteboer, M., Willems, P., Viergever, M., Niessen, W.: Brain shift estimation in image-guided neurosurgery using 3-D ultrasound. IEEE Transactions on Biomedical Engineering 52(2), 268–276 (2005)

12. Mercier, L., Fonov, V., Haegelen, C., Del Maestro, R., Petrecca, K., Collins, D.: Comparing two approaches to rigid registration of three-dimensional ultrasound and magnetic resonance images for neurosurgery. International Journal of Computer Assisted Radiology and Surgery, 1–12 (2011)

13. Otsu, N.: A threshold selection method from gray-level histograms. IEEE Transactions on Systems, Man and Cybernetics 9(1), 62–66 (1979)

14. Roche, A., Pennec, X., Malandain, G., Ayache, N.: Rigid registration of 3D ultrasound with MR images: a new approach combining intensity and gradient information. IEEE Trans. Med. Imaging 20, 1038–1049 (2001)

15. Wein, W., Brunke, S., Khamene, A., Callstrom, M.R., Navab, N.: Automatic ct-ultrasound registration for diagnostic imaging and image-guided intervention. Medical Image Analysis 12(5), 577–585 (2008)

16. Zhang, W., Noble, J., Brady, J.: Adaptive Non-rigid Registration of Real Time 3D Ultrasound to Cardiovascular MR Images. In: Karssemeijer, N., Lelieveldt, B. (eds.) IPMI 2007. LNCS, vol. 4584, pp. 50–61. Springer, Heidelberg (2007)

Atlas-Based Segmentation of the Subthalamic Nucleus, Red Nucleus, and Substantia Nigra for Deep Brain Stimulation by Incorporating Multiple MRI Contrasts

Yiming Xiao[1], Lara Bailey[1], M. Mallar Chakravarty[2,3], Silvain Beriault[1], Abbas F. Sadikot[4], G. Bruce Pike[1], and D. Louis Collins[1]

[1] Montreal Neurological Institute, McGill University, Montreal, Canada
[2] Kimel Family Translational Imaging Genetics Laboratory, The Centre for Addiction and Mental Health, Toronto, Canada
[3] Department of Psychiatry, University of Toronto, Toronto, Canada
[4] Division of Neurosurgery, McGill University, Montreal, Canada

Abstract. Deep brain stimulation (DBS) of the subthalamic nucleus (STN) is an effective therapy for drug-resistant Parkinson's disease (PD). Pre-operative identification of the STN is an important step for this neurosurgical procedure, but is very challenging because of the accuracy necessary to stimulate only a sub-region of the small STN to achieve the maximum therapeutic benefits without serious side effects. Previously, a technique that automatically identified basal ganglia structures was proposed by registering a 3D histological atlas to a subject's anatomy shown in the T1w MRI image. In this paper, we improve the accuracy of this technique for the segmentation of the STN, substantia nigra (SN), and red nucleus (RN). This is achieved by using additional MRI contrasts (i.e. T2*w and T2w images) that can better visualize these nuclei compared to the sole T1w contrast used previously. Through validation using the silver standard ground truth obtained for 6 subjects (3 healthy and 3 PD), we observe significant improvements for segmenting the STN, SN, and RN with the new technique when compared to the previous method that only uses T1w-T1w inter-subject registration.

1   Introduction

Parkinson's disease (PD) is a progressive and chronic disease of the central nervous system (CNS). Deep brain stimulation (DBS) at the dorsal-lateral site of the subthalamic nucleus (STN) is an effective treatment for relieving motor symptoms (tremor, akinesia, rigidity) of Parkinson's disease [1]. Determining the geometry of the STN is an important step before locating the motor-function region (or dorsal-lateral site) for this neuro-surgical procedure because stimulation of only this sub-region results in desirable therapeutic benefits without side effects. Yet, locating the precise stimulation target is difficult because the STN is small and is in close proximity to several delicate structures, such as the red

P. Abolmaesumi et al. (Eds.): IPCAI 2012, LNAI 7330, pp. 135–145, 2012.
© Springer-Verlag Berlin Heidelberg 2012

nucleus (RN) and the substantia nigra (SN). Many methods have been proposed previously to locate the stimulation targets [1], and are divided into direct and indirect targeting methods. Direct targeting methods [1] rely on MRI sequences that directly visualize the geometry of the STN. Among these, susceptibility-based methods (i.e. T2*w images and R2* maps) offer better contrast [2] while the T2w Fast-Spin-Echo (FSE) acquisitions are more commonly used [1]. Either way, manual identification is still necessary to determine the target stimulation site. Indirect methods often involve deformation of brain atlases [1]. These procedures need less expert supervision, but the T1w-MRI-based registration may be sub-optimal since the structures of interest are not well visualized in the T1w images, and their locations must be indirectly inferred from nearby structures that have contrast on the T1w image. In this article, we propose a framework that non-rigidly deforms a digitalized histological basal ganglia atlas to segment the STN, RN, and SN by incorporating multiple MRI contrasts to estimate the deformation field. This automatic method was validated with manual segmentations of *in vivo* MRI data acquired on a 3T scanner (Siemens Tim Trio, Erlangen, Germany), and was compared with the T1w-based method introduced previously in [3]. This improved alignment will facilitate more accurate automatic delineation of the sub-region of the STN for the DBS procedure, which requires sub-millimeter accuracy in the stimulation electrode placement.

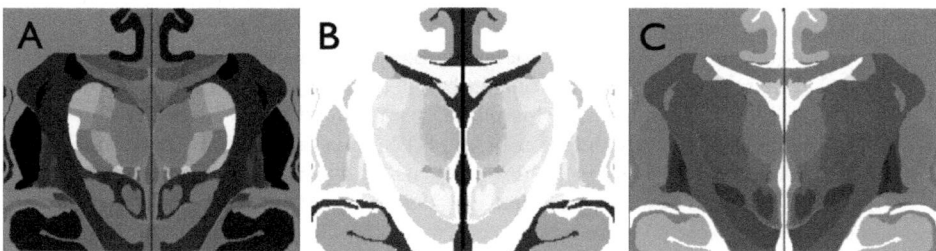

Fig. 1. A coronal view of the 3D digital basal ganglia atlas (A) and its resulting T1w pseudo-MRI (B) and T2w pseudo-MRI (C)

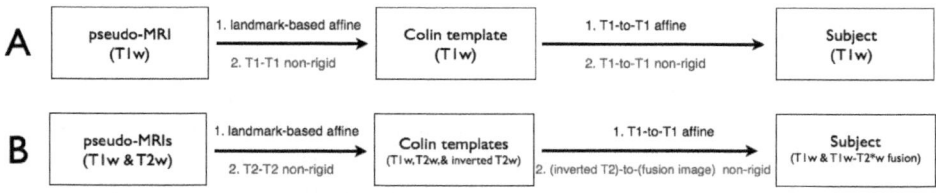

Fig. 2. Pipelines of two atlas-based segmentation schemes. A: atlas-based segmentation method with T1w-T1w registration; B: atlas-based segmentation method with multiple image contrasts incorporated. Differences between A and B are shown in red fonts.

2 Atlas-Warping Segmentation with T1w-T1w Registration

Previously, a high-resolution 3D digital basal ganglia atlas (Fig. 1A) was derived from a post-mortem healthy brain [4]. In addition, a framework to deform this atlas for segmenting basal ganglia structures on an individual's anatomy was also proposed and validated for the globus palllidus (GP), striatum, and thalamus [3]. This segmentation framework only employed T1w images, and the deformation of the basal ganglia atlas was completed in two steps using a global affine and local non-rigid registration strategy. A flow-chart demonstrating the procedure is shown in Fig. 2A. In the first step, the atlas was fitted to the T1-weighted (T1w) Colin27 brain template (Fig. 3A) [5], and this was achieved in two stages. In the first stage, the brain atlas was aligned to the Colin27 template with an affine transformation based on the estimate of 24 homologous landmarks pairs (details in [3]). These homologous landmark pairs were selected on structures well visible on the T1w images, such as the striatum, the lateral ventricle, and thalamus. In the second stage, a pseudo-MRI (Fig.1B) was created by manually assigning each atlas label the intensity value in the corresponding region of the T1w Colin27 template. Then, with ANIMAL non-linear registration [6], this T1-appearing pseudo-MRI was non-rigidly registered to the Colin27 template to further refine the fit between the atlas and the template. After the deformation, the digital brain atlas was brought into the space of Colin27 template. In the second step, the Colin27 template and the co-registered atlas were mapped to the anatomy of a subject seen on the T1w MR image. This was completed in a similar manner as the first step, except the affine transformation was completed automatically using a hierarchical approach with cross-correlation for the cost function. In [3], three variants of the atlas-to-subject registration methods were compared. Based on the segmentation quality of the T1w visible brain structures (i.e. GP, thalamus, and striatum), the strategy described above was considered to be the optimal approach. However, while this atlas-based segmentation technique is robust for

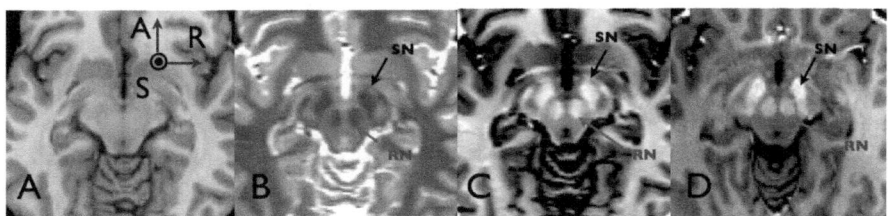

Fig. 3. Images (axial view) used in the proposed automatic nuclei segmentation framework. A=T1w Colin27 template; B=T2w Colin template; C="intensity inverted" T2w Colin template; D=T1w-T2*w fusion image of a healthy female subject. Please note that A-C are in Talairach space, and D is in the native space. The STN and RN are identified in B-D.The coordinates in Talairach space are marked in A, where A=anterior, R=right, and S=superior.

structures easily identifiable on T1w images, its segmentation performance on the STN, RN, and SN may still require further improvement due to the poor contrast of these nuclei in the T1w images, and thus their anatomical variability is not as fully accounted for as other structures (i.e. ventricles, striatum, etc.).

3   Atlas-Warping Segmentation with Multiple MRI Contrasts Registration

At present, FSE T2w MRI images are considered to be the state of the art image acquisition technique to directly visualize the nuclei, such as the STN, SN, and RN. However, the drawback lies in the long scanning times required to achieve high resolution full brain coverage (i.e. $1 \times 1 \times 1 mm^3$), and it is not perfect for DBS target planning in patients with movement disorders. In addition, the specific absorption rate (SAR) for FSE sequences is often higher than the gradient-echo (GRE) sequences. Recent developments have led to new MRI techniques for visualizing the STN. Among these, the susceptibility-based MRI methods, such as the T2*w image and R2* (1/T2*) map, have demonstrated comparable or better contrast of the STN than the FSE T2w sequences, while providing a higher resolution in a relatively clinically feasible time. We hypothesize that by incorporating the MRI techniques which can directly visualize the STN, SN, and RN into the framework introduced in the previous section, the non-rigid registration should improve the atlas-to-template warping, the template-to-subject warping, as well as the resulting atlas-to-subject warping. As a result, the overall segmentation accuracy should increase. The previous technique in [3] uses T1w-image registration only. While preserving the parameters of the global affine and local non-rigid registration strategy in [3], here we used a T2w-appearing pseudo-MRI, a T2w Colin template, an "intensity-inverted" T2w Colin template, and T1w-T2*w fusion MRI images of the subjects for the local non-rigid registration. Note that the pipeline of this new framework is illustrated in Fig. 2B. The creation the new MRI modalities and the registration procedures are detailed in the following sections.

3.1   T2w Colin MRI Template and T2w Pseudo-MRI

Since the Colin27 T1w template was not able to provide sufficient contrast for the STN and its neighboring SN and RN, a co-aligned T2w FSE Colin template and its corresponding T2w pseudo-MRI were created. First, the T2w Colin template was produced from 12 FSE T2w MR images ($1 \times 1 mm^2$ in-plane resolution, $2mm$ slice thickness in sagittal direction) of the same subject as the Colin27 T1w template ([5]). Each T2w image was processed using the following sequence: 1) rigid registration to Colin27 T1w template using normalized mutual information as the objective function [7] and resampling to the Colin27 template grid with sinc-function interpolation; 2) image intensity inhomogeneity correction [8]; 3) image intensity normalization [9]; and 4) non-local means image de-noising [10]. Lastly, the T2w Colin template (Fig. 3B) was generated by averaging these

12 pre-processed images. In this resulting T2w average template, the GP, STN, SN, and RN demonstrate their characteristic hypo-intensity features, while their boundary delineations were improved due to image averaging. The creation of the T2w pseudo-MRI (Fig. 1C) follows the same manner as the original T1w pseudo-MRI except that the intensity values were taken from the Colin T2w image instead of the Colin27 T1w image.

3.2   Inverted T2w Colin Template and T1w-T2*w Fusion Image

Ideally, one would register T2w FSE patient data with the new Colin T2w template to customize the atlas to the patient's anatomy. Unfortunately, it is difficult, if not impossible, to acquire high resolution T2w FSE in clinically acceptable times. We proposed to acquire data with a 10-echo 3D FLASH MRI sequence [11], with the following parameters: echo time (TE)=$\{1.6, 4.1, 6.6, 9.1, 13.0, 16.0, 18.5, 21.0, 23.5, 26.0\}$ms, repetition time (TR) =30 ms, flip-angle=23°, read out bandwidth=±450 Hz/pix, acquisition matrix=256x256, 176 sagittal slices, resolution=$0.95\times0.95\times0.95mm^{3}$, 6/8 partial Fourier in the phase and slice encoding directions, and GRAPPA factor =2, acquisition time = 7:05 min. From the MRI data acquired, three original image contrasts (T1w image, T2*w image, and R2* map) were generated. The T1w image was produced by averaging the magnitude images of the first four echoes. The T2*w image was generated by averaging the magnitude images of the last five echoes. The R2* map was derived by least-square fitting all magnitude data to an exponential curve. These three image contrasts are shown in Fig. 4 for a healthy female subject. Since all three image contrasts were generated in the same scan session, no inter-contrast registration is necessary. The T2*w image and R2* map were used later to establish the silver standard ground truth for evaluation. While non-linear registration of the Colin FSE T2w image and the T2*w patient image might be possible with a mutual information based cost function, we propose to use ANIMAL cross-correlation-based non-linear registration of an "intensity-inverted" T2w Colin template (Fig. 3C) and a T1w-T2*w fusion patient image (Fig. 3D). The patient's fusion image is synthesized using $I_{fusion} = I_{T1w} + (I_{T1w} - I_{T2*w} \times \alpha)$, where I_{fusion}, I_{T1w}, and I_{T2*w} represent the voxel intensities of the fusion image, T1w image, and T2*w image, respectively, and α is the normalization factor that ensures the voxel intensity of the white matter in the T2*w image is at the same level as the T1w image. Last, the "intensity-inverted" T2w Colin template is simply obtained by subtracting the intensity of the T2w Colin template from its maximum value. The use of cross-correlation objective function is justified by the similar image contrast of the two synthesized images (Fig. 3C and 3D), and enables direct comparison with the previous T1w-T1w technique [3].

3.3   Atlas-to-Subject Registration

As shown in Fig. 2B, the new multi-contrast atlas-based customization procedure was completed in two steps. In the first step, the atlas was fitted to the Colin templates. This was done in two stages: First, the previously computed

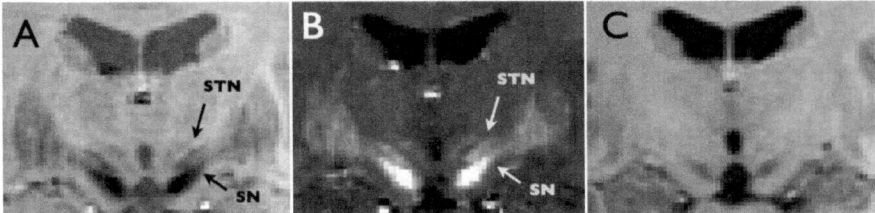

Fig. 4. Coronal slices of T2*w image (A), R2* map (B), and T1w image (C) obtained from the 10 echo 3D FLASH sequences for a healthy female subject. The STN and SN are identified in A and B, but are poorly visualized in C.

landmark-based affine registration [3] brought the atlas roughly to the space of Colin27; Second, local non-rigid registration (in the region of the basal ganglia) was used to fine-tune the remaining anatomical differences between the atlas and Colin27. This step was performed by deforming the T2w basal ganglia pseudo-MRI to the T2w Colin MRI template. In the second half of the pipeline, the Colin template anatomy was brought into each individual's anatomy in two stages. First, an affine registration between the T1w Colin27 template and a subject's T1w image was performed. Susceptibility artifacts (signal drop-outs near the sinus, orbitofrontal and temporal lobes) exist for T2*w MRI, but not for T2w or T1w MRI. Thus, the fusion image has unwanted artifacts near the cortical surface, and for the global affine registration, we think T1-T1 registration is a sufficient and better choice. The "intensity-inverted" T2w Colin template, co-registered with the Colin27 template, was then warped to the T1w-T2*w fusion image of the subject through a local non-rigid registration procedure. Finally, the digital brain atlas was warped using the recovered transformations to the designated subject's anatomy in order to segment the basal ganglia. In the entire pipeline, the registration parameters remained the same as the original T1w-image only framework [3]. Although it is possible to achieve the non-rigid registration by considering a pair of MRIs (T1w and an additional contrast) simultaneously, we feel that using the T2w and fusion images alone is sufficient since the structural information in T1w images is still included in these images for the region of interest, and pair-wise multi-contrast registration is computationally more expensive.

4   Evaluation

4.1   Subjects and Establishment of Ground Truth

After providing informed consent, 3 healthy subjects (1 female, 2 male, age= 37 ± 12 yr) and 3 PD patients (1 female, 2 male, age=54 ± 4 yr) volunteered for the study. Each subject was scanned with the proposed 10-echo 3D FLASH MRI sequence. From the acquired MRI data, the T1w image, T2*w image, R2* map, and T1w-T2*w fusion image were produced for each subject. Two sets of silver standard ground truth for the STN, SN, and RN were made by one expert's manual identification on the MRI images: 1. ground truth for Colin (called "**GT1**"); 2. ground truth for each testing subject (called "**GT2**"). The first set was used to examine the quality of atlas-to-template registration, and the second set was applied to validate the quality of the template-to-subject registration, as well as the segmentation performance of the entire system for the STN, RN, and SN. With ITK-SNAP (www.itkSNAP.org), we obtained the ground truth for the Colin template by manually painting the labels of the STN, SN, and RN on the T2w Colin template in 3D. For all 6 subjects, the manual labels were painted using a consensus of the patient's T2*w image and R2* map.

4.2   Evaluation Methods

In total, three aspects of the final atlas-warping pipeline were examined with respect to segmenting the STN, SN, and RN: 1. quality of atlas-to-template registration; 2. quality of template-to-subject registration; 3. the segmentation performance of the entire system for the nuclei of interest. For the atlas-to-template registration, we compared the Colin27-coregistered histological atlas with the manual segmentation of T2w Colin template ("**GT1**"); In the second aspect, "**GT1**" was employed as an atlas label set and warped to a subject's anatomy with the deformation matrix obtained in the second half of the pipeline, then compared to "**GT2**" in the native space of each subject. Last, the deformed histological atlas was compared with the manually painted labels of each subject ("**GT2**"). For each test, three evaluation metrics were computed to compared the warped labels and the ground truth: 1) the overlap metric **kappa=2*a/(b+c)**, where **a** is the intersection of two segmentations, and **b** and **c** are volumes of each segmentation; 2) the Euclidean distance (COM_{Euclid}) between the centre of mass (COM) of the deformed labels and the silver standard ground truth; and 3) the COM coordinate differences ($\Delta COM_{R,A,S} = COM_{atlas}\text{-}COM_{ground-truth}$) after transforming them into the Talairach space (the coordinates are shown in Fig. 3A). The evaluation results were analyzed using one-sample or paired-sample one-sided t-tests. In the next section, we compared all these metrics for both the original T1w-image-only pipeline, and the newly proposed pipeline with multiple image contrasts added.

4.3   Results

A qualitative examination was conducted between the warped-atlases and the manually identified ground truth for both Colin and the 6 testing subjects. Figure 5 shows coronal views of the warped labels and the manual segmentation of the SN, STN, and RN, overlaid on Colin's and a healthy subject's T1w images. In Fig. 5, the first row (Fig. 5B, 5D, and 5F) shows the result of the registration method in [3]; the second row (Fig. 5C, 5E, and 5G) demonstrates the results of our updated registration framework. From the visual inspection, we are able to see the warped labels in the second row demonstrate higher resemblance with the ground truths for both Colin (**GT1**) and the subject (**GT2**).

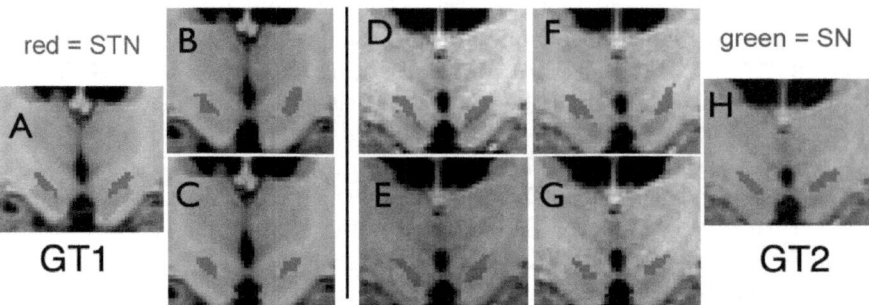

Fig. 5. Results of atlas registration and the silver standard ground truth. A=**GT1**, H=**GT2**. B, D and F are segmentation results of atlas-to-template registration, template-to-subject registration, and complete system, respectively, by using only T1w-T1w registration. C, E and G are segmentation results of atlas-to-template registration, template-to-subject registration, and complete system, respectively, by using multiple image contrasts. Please note that to the **left** of the black line, Image A, B, and C show the labels of Colin; to the **right** side, labels are shown for a healthy female subject.

The quantitative differences between the method in [3] and our updated technique for atlas-to-template registration, template-to-subject registration, and segmentation performance of the complete system, are listed in Table 1, 2, and 3, respectively.

Comparing the results obtained by the two procedures, in general, our new method improves the two registration stages (atlas-to-template and template-to-subject), as well as the segmentation performance of the overall system. For the atlas-to-template registration, improvements are seen for the three metrics for RN and STN. For the SN, while the kappa value increased, the distance

Table 1. Evaluation of atlas-to-template registration. The results of T1w registration are shown in **bold black**, and results of our multi-contrast method are shown in blue. For $\Delta COM_{R,A,S}$, R, A, and S represent the right, anterior, and superior-directions respectively in Talairach space. The same formatting applies to Table 2 and 3.

Side	Metric	RN			SN			STN		
Left	**kappa**	**0.39**			**0.45**			**0.52**		
		0.83			0.56			0.71		
	COM_{Euclid} (mm)	**3.14**			**3.51**			**2.41**		
		0.40			3.87			0.35		
		R	A	S	R	A	S	R	A	S
	$\Delta COM_{R,A,S}$ (mm)	**-0.85**	**2.30**	**1.97**	**1.45**	**-3.20**	**0.09**	**-1.74**	**0.70**	**1.51**
		-0.38	0.12	0.07	1.53	-3.09	-1.74	0.00	-0.12	0.33
Right	**kappa**	**0.43**			**0.50**			**0.42**		
		0.79			0.60			0.67		
	COM_{Euclid} (mm)	**3.09**			**3.36**			**3.15**		
		0.38			3.60			0.57		
		R	A	S	R	A	S	R	A	S
	$\Delta COM_{R,A,S}$ (mm)	**1.70**	**1.17**	**2.30**	**-1.07**	**-3.18**	**0.12**	**1.75**	**0.10**	**2.62**
		0.32	0.19	0.03	-1.35	-2.74	-1.92	-0.01	0.19	0.54

Table 2. Evaluation of template-to-subject registration

Side	Metric	RN			SN			STN		
Left	kappa	**0.72±0.05** 0.77±0.03			**0.56±0.06** 0.64±0.03			**0.55±0.08** 0.62±0.04		
	COM_{Euclid} (mm)	**1.12±0.39** 0.66±0.13			**2.42±0.56** 1.90±0.63			**1.42±0.63** 1.30±0.13		
		R	A	S	R	A	S	R	A	S
	$\Delta COM_{R,A,S}$ (mm)	**0.31** **±0.51** 0.37 ±0.18	**-0.87** **±0.50** -0.35 ±0.23	**-0.50** **±0.19** -0.31 ±0.29	**0.38** **±0.55** 0.05 ±0.47	**1.95** **±1.34** 1.57 ±1.18	**-0.79** **±0.42** -0.19 ±0.42	**0.26** **±0.64** 0.35 ±0.58	**-0.86** **±1.04** -0.52 ±0.72	**-0.50** **±0.65** -0.85 ±0.21
Right	kappa	**0.72±0.07** 0.77±0.04			**0.58±0.10** 0.68±0.05			**0.52±0.08** 0.62±0.06		
	COM_{Euclid} (mm)	**0.92±0.39** 0.40±0.18			**1.99±0.77** 1.74±1.03			**1.52±0.63** 1.04±0.63		
		R	A	S	R	A	S	R	A	S
	$\Delta COM_{R,A,S}$ (mm)	**-0.19** **±0.74** -0.36 ±0.17	**-0.48** **±0.27** -0.10 ±0.20	**-0.49** **±0.26** 0.05 ±0.10	**0.16** **±0.33** 0.12 ±0.33	**1.62** **±1.30** 1.59 ±1.38	**-0.75** **±0.23** -0.02 ±0.26	**0.32** **±1.05** 0.17 ±0.72	**-0.34** **±0.98** -0.14 ±0.68	**-0.69** **±0.48** -0.41 ±0.61

Table 3. Evaluation of the segmentation performance of the overall system

Side	Metric	RN			SN			STN		
Left	kappa	**0.54±0.06** 0.82±0.01			**0.55±0.08** 0.59±0.07			**0.56±0.08** 0.63±0.06		
	COM_{Euclid} (mm)	**1.85±0.22** 0.43±0.12			**2.54±1.33** 3.39±1.23			**1.58±0.64** 1.08±0.18		
		R	A	S	R	A	S	R	A	S
	$\Delta COM_{R,A,S}$ (mm)	**-0.23** **±0.55** -0.02 ±0.20	**1.58** **±0.15** -0.30 ±0.18	**1.00** **±0.18** -0.18 ±0.21	**1.71** **±0.64** 2.02 ±0.42	**-1.95** **±1.16** -2.02 ±1.07	**-0.53** **±0.45** -2.04 ±0.59	**-1.22** **±0.51** 0.38 ±0.58	**-0.19** **±0.98** -0.49 ±0.55	**0.60** **±0.53** -0.52 ±0.37
Right	kappa	**0.52±0.13** 0.84±0.03			**0.59±0.04** 0.57±0.06			**0.43±0.16** 0.61±0.06		
	COM_{Euclid} (mm)	**2.28±0.62** 0.26±0.09			**1.90±1.14** 3.01±0.68			**2.52±0.80** 0.94±0.44		
		R	A	S	R	A	S	R	A	S
	$\Delta COM_{R,A,S}$ (mm)	**1.56** **±0.80** -0.01 ±0.18	**0.95** **±0.20** 0.09 ±0.15	**1.53** **±0.30** -0.07 ±0.14	**-0.81** **±0.48** -1.38 ±0.42	**-1.55** **±1.12** -1.63 ±1.03	**-0.32** **±0.37** -2.09 ±0.32	**1.84** **±1.13** 0.32 ±0.69	**0.43** **±0.87** -0.08 ±0.69	**1.52** **±0.34** -0.09 ±0.52

measures didn't demonstrate improvements. For the template-to-subject registration, the improvement is significant ($p<0.05$) for the kappa metrics (SN, left RN, and right STN) and COM_{Euclid} (RN and left SN). For the segmentation of the complete system, the enhancement in segmentation performance is significant for the kappa metrics (STN, RN, and left SN), and COM_{Euclid} (RN and right STN). The COM_{Euclid} of the STN (Left:1.08±0.18 mm, Right:0.94±0.44 mm) is in the same range or better than those previously reported [1]. From the analysis of $\Delta COM_{R,A,S}$, we observed a systematic location bias in the warped atlas when using only T1w-T1w inter-subject non-rigid registration: for the template-to-subject registration, the warped labels are more posterior and inferior for the RN ($p<0.05$), and more anterior and inferior for the SN ($p<0.05$). For the complete system, the segmentations are more lateral and superior for the STN, more medial and posterior for the SN ($p<0.05$), and more anterior and superior for the RN ($p<0.05$). However, with our method, the final segmentation results of the entire system show almost no significant displacement for the RN; although the segmented left STN is more inferior ($p<0.05$), the absolute mean displacement is less than using the old method.

5 Discussion

For the SN segmentation after adding multiple MRI contrasts, the average Euclidean distance between the COMs increased while the kappa metrics improved. Since the mean Hausdorff distance of the SN between the manual and automatic segmentation is smaller with our method (Left: 6.11mm; Right: 5.63mm) than with the T1w registration (Left: 6.72mm; Right: 6.19mm), this can be explained by a tighter fit of our method to the ground truth segmentation, except at the inferior borders of the SN. Judging from Table 1 and 2, this could be due to the individual variability of the histological data, or the fact that the MRI does not reveal equal amounts of tissue as shown in chemically stained histological data. Compared with the histological atlas, the limited accuracy of manual segmentation (intra- and inter-rater variability) can only make the MRI-based atlas a silver standard due to the limits of current MRI (i.e. resolution and partial volume effect). Although label fusion techniques, together with high field MRI (i.e. 7T) may mitigate these drawbacks, ultimately the extents of the nuclei are confirmed by intra-surgical electro-physiological recording. Due to the fact that the STN is much smaller than the other structures of the basal ganglia (i.e. GP or striatum), and the image resolution is on the scale of 1 mm^3, the kappa metric may not be perfectly appropriate to represent the full potential of this new technique. There are very few previous studies evaluating volumetric segmentation of the STN, RN, and SN with overlap metrics; most report 3D distance measures only. Upon consideration of the Euclidean distances between the automatic and manual segmentation and visual inspection, our segmentation quality is satisfactory. However, efforts could still be made to further improve the system in the future. First, although the FSE T2w image and T2*w images demonstrate similar contrast in the basal ganglia system, we would like to construct multimodality templates that include both T1w and T2*w images for both healthy and PD brains in different age groups. This way, the variability in shape and in the nuclei contrasts due to aging or pathological changes can be better accounted for. Second, we believe that by adding geometric shape constraints and other image contrasts (i.e. quantitative susceptibility map), the segmentation accuracy could be enhanced. Last, we would like to compare the location of the segmented STN with electro-physiological recording to confirm its efficiency.

6 Conclusion

Upon visual inspection of the registered results using the original T1w-image-only framework, there was a coarse correspondence of the STN, SN, and RN between the warped atlas and the manual segmentations, but the geometric description is not sufficiently accurate according to the quantitative evaluation.

After incorporating MRI techniques that are capable of directly visualizing the STN and its adjacent SN and RN, we observed large improvements in separate stages of the atlas-based segmentation pipeline, as well as the segmentation performance of the entire system. This proved our original assumption that inter-subject (atlas-to-template or template-to-subject) registration with only T1w images is not sufficient for structures that are almost invisible on the T1w images, as far as the registration framework in [3] is concerned. In conclusion, we established a technique that automatically segments the STN, SN, and RN for STN deep brain stimulation, by combining MRI techniques that can directly delineate these nuclei, and a high resolution basal ganglia atlas that was defined from histological data. This framework was validated on 6 subjects (3 healthy and 3 PD patients), and is an improvement compared with the technique in [3].

References

[1] Brunenberg, E.J., Platel, B., Hofman, P.A., Ter Haar Romeny, B.M., Visser-Vandewalle, V.: Magnetic resonance imaging techniques for visualization of the subthalamic nucleus. J. Neurosurg. 115(5), 971–984 (2011)

[2] O'Gorman, R.L., Shmueli, K., Ashkan, K., Samuel, M., Lythgoe, D.J., Shahidiani, A., Jarosz, J.: Optimal MRI methods for direct stereotactic targeting of the subthalamic nucleus and globus pallidus. Eur. Radiol. 21(1), 130–136 (2011)

[3] Chakravarty, M.M., Sadikot, A.F., Germann, J., Bertrand, G., Collins, D.L.: Towards a validation of atlas warping techniques. Med. Image Anal. 12(6), 713–726 (2008)

[4] Chakravarty, M.M., Bertrand, G., Hodge, C.P., Sadikot, A.F., Collins, D.L.: The creation of a brain atlas for image guided neurosurgery using serial histological data. Neuroimage 30(2), 359–376 (2006)

[5] Holmes, C.J., Hoge, R., Collins, L., Woods, R., Toga, A.W., Evans, A.C.: Enhancement of MR images using registration for signal averaging. J. Comput. Assist. Tomogr. 22(2), 324–333 (1998)

[6] Collins, D.L., Evans, A.C.: Animal: Validation and applications of nonlinear registration-based segmentation. Int. J. Pattern Recogn. 11(8), 1271–1294 (1997)

[7] Studholme, C., Hill, D.L.G., Hawkes, D.J.: An overlap invariant entropy measure of 3D medical image alignment. Pattern Recogn. 32(1), 71–86 (1999)

[8] Sled, J.G., Zijdenbos, A.P., Evans, A.C.: A nonparametric method for automatic correction of intensity nonuniformity in MRI data. IEEE Trans. Med. Imaging 17(1), 87–97 (1998)

[9] Nyul, L.G., Udupa, J.K., Zhang, X.: New variants of a method of MRI scale standardization. IEEE Trans. Med. Imaging 19(2), 143–150 (2000)

[10] Coupé, P., Yger, P., Barillot, C.: Fast Non Local Means Denoising for 3D MR Images. In: Larsen, R., Nielsen, M., Sporring, J. (eds.) MICCAI 2006. LNCS, vol. 4191, pp. 33–40. Springer, Heidelberg (2006)

[11] Xiao, Y., Beriault, S., Pike, B.G., Collins, D.L.: Multi-contrast multi-echo FLASH MRI for targeting the subthalamic nucleus. Magn. Reson. Imaging (to appear)

Towards Systematic Usability Evaluations for the OR: An Introduction to OR-Use Framework

Ali Bigdelou, Aslı Okur, Max-Emanuel Hoffmann,
Bamshad Azizi, and Nassir Navab

Chair for Computer Aided Medical Procedures (CAMP), TU Munich, Germany

Abstract. It has been shown that usability of intra-operative computer-based systems has a direct impact on patient outcome and patient safety. There are several tools to facilitate the usability testing in other domains, however, there is no such tool for the operating room. In this work, after investigating the features of the existing tools in other domains and observing the practical requirements specific to the OR, we summarize key functionalities that should be provided in a usability testing support tool for intra-operative devices. Furthermore, we introduce the OR-Use framework, a tool developed for supporting usability evaluation for the OR and designed to fulfill the introduced requirements. Finally, we report about several performed tests to evaluate the performance of the proposed framework. We also report about the usability tests which have been conducted up until now using this tool.

1 Introduction

Computer-based systems in the Operating Rooms (OR) have become widely used as a means of improving the treatment process and the patient outcome. On the other hand, this can increase the risks for human error. According to a study published in 2004 [12], between 44,000 to 98,000 patients die each year from preventable medical errors in American hospitals where 69% of these events are rooted in wrong usage of technical equipment. This problem can be targeted by studying the usability of intra-operative devices. Usability can be defined by the ease with which a user can operate, prepare inputs for, and interpret outputs of a system or component. Nielsen states that usability is associated with five main attributes: Learnability, Efficiency, Memorability, Errors, and Satisfaction [10]. This definition has been extended within different industrial standards for certain contexts, e.g. ISO IEC 62366 for the medical domain. Among available usability evaluation approaches, Liljegren [7] suggested that usability testing is more appropriate for medical devices. It consists of four main stages as planning, conducting, analysis and report. Performing a complete usability test is not always an easy endeavor due to many challenges associated with the acquisition and the management of usability data as well as the analysis of huge amount of collected information. In order to overcome these challenges, several usability

P. Abolmaesumi et al. (Eds.): IPCAI 2012, LNAI 7330, pp. 146–156, 2012.

evaluation support tools have been proposed in different domains as reported by Ivory and Hearst [6]. Such tools reduce the required amount of labour and costs assigned to these tests and therefore they can be performed on a frequent, iterative basis, within the development life-cycle. Despite its vital effect, to our knowledge, there is no such support tool for the OR domain and usability study is often neglected due to its complexity and relatively high demand of time and resources. Furthermore, none of the previous frameworks are considering the complexities of the OR, hence making them impractical in this context.

The complex nature of the OR domain makes the production of usable intra-operative devices very challenging. The OR is a collaborative environment where multiple potential users perform together, each with different individual roles e.g. surgeon, nurse. Usually, intra-operative devices are targeting more than one of these roles and therefore their usability should be studied for each individual target role. Additionally, the usages of intra-operative devices are usually fused in activities of a higher level process model known as surgical workflow [9]. In this situation, defining atomic test tasks as it is done for websites or handheld devices is not practical. Moreover, the intra-operative devices are technically much more advanced compared to web sites. They are often compose of additional external hardware such as probes and tracking systems, which are integrated as part of their user interface (UI). Taking into account that interaction with all these external parts of the UI should be also considered within the usability test, the challenges facing the usability specialist in this domain become clear. In [4], we proposed a conceptual model for managing the usability data. This model decomposes the complexities of the OR domain into three views as surgical workflow, human roles and intra-operative device, where cross-view correlations are stored in mapping tables. In this work, we propose the main functionalities required for a usability testing support tool and explain a possible architecture for exploiting models similar to the one proposed in [4] for supporting intra-operative usability testing. Finally, we conclude with a comparison with similar tools and report about our early results from conducted experiments.

1.1 Related Works

There are many tools and frameworks to support usability testing in different domains. Morae [8], Mangold INTERACT and Nodlus Observer are commercially available tools which consist of a recorder and analysis tools. Several tools are further introduced for usability studies of web-based applications such as Web Usability Probe [1]. Technically, they analyze the html source of the web pages and by adding a spy script for each UI control, generate a usage report. Similarly, authors in [3] propose HUIA framework to record and visualize the interaction logs for applications on smart phones. Furthermore, SAVE [5] provides comparable functionalities for augmented reality applications where users interact in a virtual environment. During the analysis stage the recorded data can be played back in the virtual scene, providing interaction information in the same fashion as the recorded videos. In the OR context, there are several methodological studies available on the topic [11]. However, no specialized support tool has been proposed until now. The closest work to our approach is presented by authors in [9] to record surgical workflows. This is a valuable tool to monitor activities within a surgical intervention; however it is not intended to be used for usability studies and does not record any user feedback or interaction logs.

2   Usability Testing for the OR

In this work, we take example of usability study of an intra-operative imaging device, incorporating a navigated handheld gamma probe. This study has been conducted in collaboration with the manufacturer. We present three case studies to highlight some of the issues about the usability of intra-operative devices.

Subjective Satisfaction. This refers to how pleasant users find it to use a system. This is an important measure since it helps to improve the user experience in order to increase customer acceptance. It is mainly evaluated based on heuristic feedback collected from test subjects. As opposed to typical scenarios such as websites, where there is one user working with the system, in the OR this should be evaluated separately for each potential human role. Presenting this information based on different aspects of the OR domain, e.g. workflow stages, it would be possible to prioritize the required improvement based on them.

Learnability per Human Role. Learnability can be defined as a measure of the degree to which interaction with a device can be learned quickly and effectively. It can be measured either with time or comparing number of performed interactions of new users to an optimum set performed by an expert user, accomplishing the very same task. In collaborative environments such as OR, this should be measured for each individual role. Smooth integration and reduced training cost are among the main benefits of a learnable system.

Cross Configurations Efficiency Comparison. In context of iterative evaluations, it is very important to compare the efficiency of the two successive versions. A system is called efficient when a user can use it productively with a minimum amount of resources such as time. One of the most common techniques for evaluating efficiency is measuring the task completion time. This may be achieved using instances running on different locations within multi-center studies.

3   Functionalities

We summarize the requirements of a usability testing support tool based on observations made with medical industry and features available in existing tools.

Planning. This is the first step of usability testing and usability support tools in this context should provide the specialist with a proper modeling technique for defining the domain model. For the OR Scenario this includes: (1) *Workflow model* which explains the sequence of activities during a surgical intervention. Having this model, the user interactions can be associated to corresponding stage within the operation. (2) *Human roles* which define different actors within a given surgical intervention. Modeling the OR roles helps to understand the usability measures from the perspective of different users. (3) *Device model* which contains all the features in a system's interface that user can interact with, such as UI controls or handheld probes. This model helps to track the user interactions.

Conducting. During this stage, a wide range of information is synchronously recorded such as: (1) *Video recording*, which is the most common technique in usability testing as it can be used to find out about the effort users make accomplishing a given task. (2) *Performance logging*, which is storing all the users' interactions with different features of the interface. Excessive amounts of clicks, scrolling and probe movements, are possible indicators for poor efficiency. (3) *Recording annotations*, which provides a great insight into the real feelings and comments of the users about the system. A dedicated tool can facilitate this and furthermore be utilized for labeling the start and end of workflow stages. Portability and easy deployment are among the main characteristics of such a tool [9], due to the fact that the monitored surgeries usually take place in different ORs, often with a very short notice. Using a portable device satisfies these needs, however, this tool itself should be highly usable due to time constraints during surgery. Small display size and limited interaction possibilities are among the main challenges for designing an annotation tool for small portable devices like smart phones. (4) *Configuration management*, which includes software and hardware version, test location and date as well as the information about the surgical team such as level of experience. This information provides the required background for analysis of multi-center and cross-configuration tests.

Analysis. Large sets of collected usability data are rarely explanatory on their own and should be analyzed for making conclusions. Several functionalities can be provided to assist the analysis process: (1) *Data retrieval*, which is a fundamental part of many usability support tools that provides a way for searching, filtering and retrieving a subset of the collected usability data. Different aspects of the domain model can be used to filter the data. (2) *Video indexing*, which provides a mean to retrieve the corresponding video segments for each piece of usability data such as user comments or performance logs. This facilitates the analysis stage by reducing the required time for browsing the videos. (3) *Visualization*, including graphs and other diagrams, which should be used where possible to draw attention to the critical issues. These can significantly reduce the time required for exploration and decision making processes.

4   OR-Use Framework

In this section we describe the architecture and main components of the OR-Use framework, shown in Figure 1 (a), developed to achieve the above mentioned requirements. According to the classification of Ivory and Hearst [6], the OR-Use framework solution for usability testing involves: capturing logs generated at client-side and storing them on the server-side, supporting analysis and a number of visualizations to ease the identification of the usability issues, and can

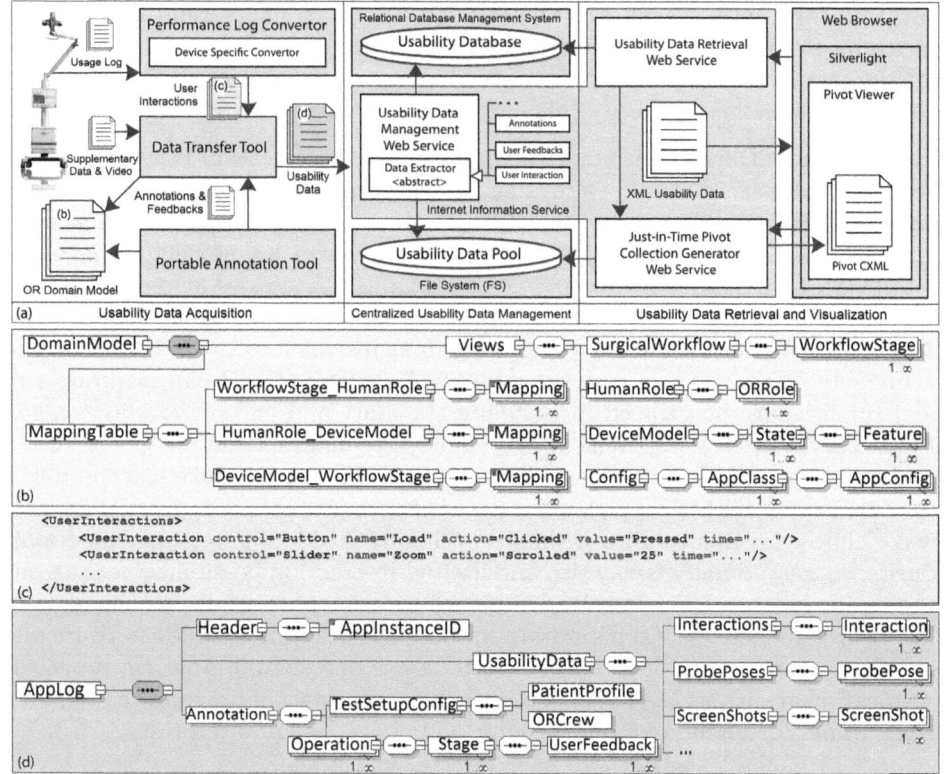

Fig. 1. Architecture of the OR-Use framework and proposed data schema

be used both for test tasks and real usage of the device. In this work we have exploited the modeling technique presented in [4]. Three views of the surgical workflow, human roles, devices and their mapping are defined in an XML file, in the planning phase. Figure 1 (b) demonstrates the schema of this XML file. Different parts of the OR-Use framework use this file as settings for initialization.

4.1 Usability Data Acquisition

In order to collect information during the usability tests, two different tools are provided. Additional to the collected data with these tools, captured video and other device specific files can be attached to the usability data. The timing is synchronized among different modules using an online time web service.

Performance Log Conversion Tool. Wide range of technologies is being used by producers of intra-operative devices, which often varies widely based on their specific requirements. In order to stay independent and extend the functional domain of the OR-Use framework, a conversion kernel is developed to convert the logs generated by a specific device to a uniform XML representation. For

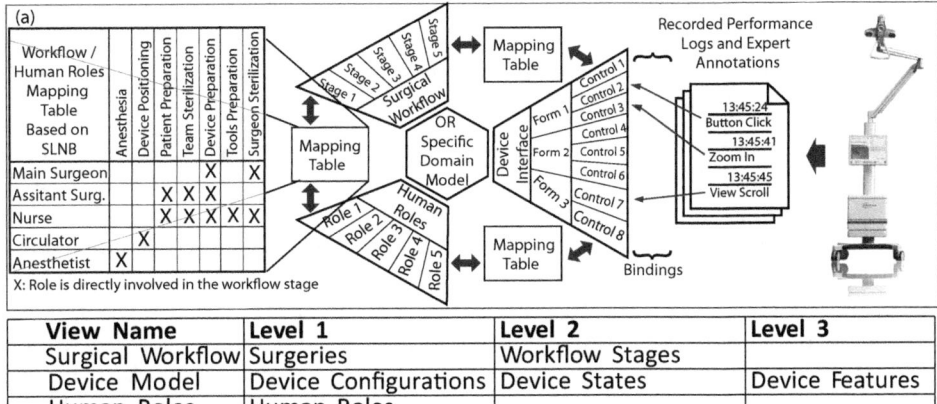

Fig. 2. (a) Structuring the usability data, (b) Relational database tables

each new device, a component can be provided and added to the conversion kernel. As shown in Figure 1 (c) the performance log XML file consists of a list of interactions. After each test session this tool is used to export the device performance logs.

Portable Annotation Tool. A portable annotation tool is developed for Android smart phone devices. This tool facilitates onsite documentations of specialist's observations. Before starting the test, for each member of the surgical team a test subject profile can be either defined or selected among the previously stored profiles. This profile contains information such as name, role and level of experience. Furthermore, during the surgery this tool is used to follow the surgical workflow stages as defined in the domain model. For each workflow stage, a button is automatically generated on the workflow page and can be used to annotate its start during the intervention. Within each workflow stage, comments can be added in two different ways: typing or voice recording. Additionally the type of OR members' comments, such as complaints or positive feedback can be specified. After the operation, all the recorded data is exported in an XML file.

4.2 Centralized Usability Data Management

For supporting cross configuration and multi-center usability studies, the OR-Use framework has been designed based on client-server architecture, as shown in Figure 1 (a). All the captured data are transferred to a server, hosting this information. Here we explain relevant components of this design.

Data Transfer. A client-side tool is developed to facilitate the uploading process. This application merges and encrypts different generated XML files, performance logs and test annotations, into a single XML message. The structure of this XML message is shown in Figure 1 (d). Multiple instances of this tool can be used simultaneously. Since the message contains all the required information about the test setup configuration, it can facilitate evaluation of different devices with different configurations conducted in various locations and hospitals.

Server Side Extraction. On the server side, the received data are decrypted, extracted and stored on the server. Each part of the XML message is processed with a corresponding data extractor component, loaded at runtime. Data extractors parse the XML data and store them in the corresponding tables of a database. Supplementary materials are separately stored on the local file system of the server, forming a repository named data pool. Each extractor component is developed for processing a special type of data, e.g. user interactions or probe readings. Such an open architecture allows the proposed framework to be extended for new devices and makes it applicable for different usability standards.

Data Management. Retrieved data on the server side is stored in a relational database. As shown in Figure 2 (a), a hierarchical representation is used in each view [4]. The depth of this hierarchy depends on level of granularity required and is defined in the domain model file. As shown in Figure 2 (b), a table is created in the database for each level of this hierarchical representation. A foreign key is used to specify the relation to the parent of each node. Usability data are separately stored, each in a dedicated table such as interactions, comments, etc.

4.3 Usability Data Retrieval and Visualization

Two web services have been developed, to access the stored usability data on the OR-Use server either directly (low-level approach) or using visualization (high-level approach). The web-based nature of these services allows multiple and simultaneous access to the data, which is important for comparison.

Usability Data Retrieval Interface. The stored usability data on the OR-Use server can be retrieved in form of XML, from standard web browsers, sending a query to a data retrieval web service, shown in Figure 1 (a). This query contains a set of key and value pairs, which are used to filter the retrieved results. The first key is *collection*, which specifies the usability data type. For all the database tables shown in Figure 2 (b), a key with similar name is defined. On the data retrieval service, this query is parsed and a SQL command is generated and executed against the database. The retrieved results are then returned as XML, which can be used for the development of additional analysis support tools such as data visualization or data mining. For example, the following query allows the usability engineer to retrieve the interactions that the surgeon has done with the brightness slider, during the scanning stage, on version 2.3 of the device:

```
HostAddress?collection="UserInteraction"&Configuration="2_3"&Workf
lowStage="Scanning"&HumanRole="Surgeon"&DeviceFeature="Brightness"
```

Usability Data Visualization. A high level visualization of the usability data can facilitate the analysis process by reducing the analyzing time. Such interface has been developed, using Microsoft Pivot and CXML file, which is an XML file

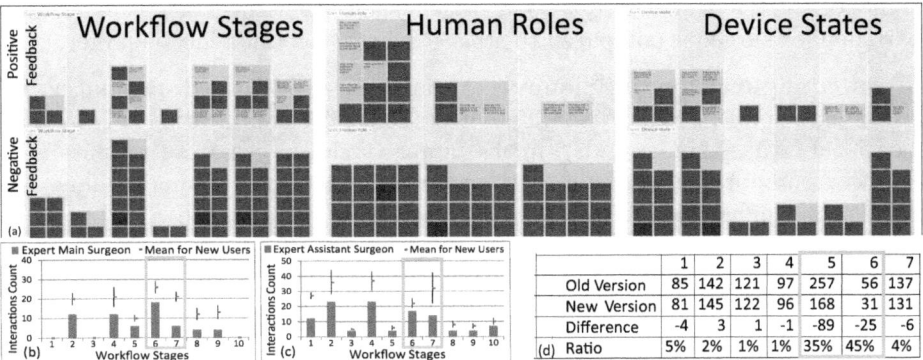

Fig. 3. Results for case studies: a)Satisfaction, b-c)Learnability, d)Efficiency

expressing a collection of items and their properties. A web service is developed to generate the CXML files using "Just-in-Time" method that makes it possible to dynamically produce collections, based on the user request. Same format as data retrieval interface is used for queries. The Pivot web service generates the CXML file based on the retrieved results from the data retrieval interface. Facets are assigned to each item based on the available information in the corresponding table and additionally other properties traceable via mappings. An image is generated per item, which simply represents its content e.g. user comments are shown as texts with a background color assigned based on their type. Also, a proper segment of the recorded video is extracted and attached, using the time of the usability data item. This is equivalent to typical video indexing.

5   Case Studies

Until the middle of November 2011, the OR-Use is used to conduct usability tests in 12 user studies and 7 surgeries took place in our partner university hospital. 5 surgeons and 10 biomedical students were involved as test subjects. A surgical workflow was modeled with 18 stages and 5 main intra-operative human roles were defined. The device modeled with 122 features in 12 stages. Within 85 performed workflow stages, about 2000 user interactions and 163 user feedbacks, annotated with one of 8 comment types have been collected, using thinking allowed. Here we report on the results for the given case studies.

Subjective satisfaction is evaluated using direct feedbacks received from the users through thinking aloud process. Figure 3 (a) shows these feedbacks, presented based on surgical workflow, human roles and device states.

Learnability per human role has been evaluated by comparing the number of interactions, required to accomplish a given task, between an expert user and new users. Figure 3 (b-c) shows these results per human role, distributed over different workflow stages. Several points can be highlighted, e.g. the close results of an expert and new users in stage 6 shows that this stage is much more learnable for surgeons compared to stage 7 where this difference is larger.

Cross configurations efficiency comparison is performed, computing the task completion time using two different versions of the application. Figure 3 (d) shows these times (in seconds), in the newer version a visualization parameter has been computed automatically, removing the need for manual tuning. The difference is higher in stages where this feature is used (5 and 6).

6 Framework Evaluation

The effectiveness of some existing tools which are used in other domains is examined and compared to the OR-Use framework. Figure 4 (d) demonstrates how well each tool meets the functional requirements, discussed in Section 3. In order to evaluate the performance of the proposed client-server architecture, we have measured the uploading and processing time with data of 30, 60 and 90 MB size, as shown in Figure 4 (a), running on a 2.5 GHz Intel Core 2 Duo machine with 4 GB of memory connected via a shared wireless network. This data was collected in 3 different test sessions, lasting about 15 minutes. Moreover, we measured the uploading and processing times when several clients simultaneously accessed the server, uploading data of 100 MB size, as shown in Figure 4 (b).

These diagrams demonstrate that by increasing the size of data and the number of clients, the processing time does not change as much as the uploading time. This means that the main bottleneck of the whole process is the uploading phase and it highlights the importance of the bandwidth in a larger setup. Also, to evaluate the usability of the proposed portable annotation tool, we conducted an ad-

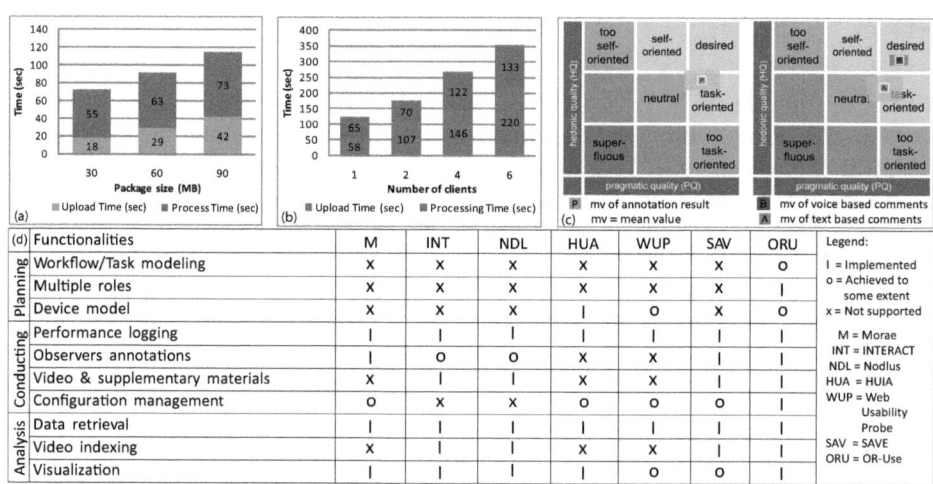

Fig. 4. OR-Use a-b)Performance evaluation, c)Usability study, d)Comparison

ditional user study with 12 participants (biomedical students aged 22 to 32). After performing a set of tasks based on real activities that a usability specialist should perform during an operation, users were asked to fill three AttrakDiff [2] questionnaires. One about profile management and workflow follow up functionalities and two about the two alternate methods for documenting the user feedbacks. The results, shown in Figure 4 (c), which place this tool in terms of pragmatic quality (PQ) and hedonic quality (HQ). PQ addresses different aspects of human needs and usability factors related to control, learnability and ease of use. HQ deals with human desires for excitement, including novelty and satisfaction. The profile management and workflow follow-up is categorized as "Task-Oriented". High PQ value means that these features have high usability factors. The large confidence area in both dimensions highlights the fact that users had diverse ideas about these features. Furthermore, keyboard-based and voice-based feedback documentation methods have been compared, where the latter is rated as more usable and interesting for intra-operative usability studies.

7   Conclusion

Usability is very important for intra-operative devices, because those with poor usability can increase the chance of human error. Having a tool for supporting different aspects of usability testing can increase testing efficiency and improve the usability of intra-operative devices. Ideally, usability testing support tools should capture a wide range of inputs, manage and organize the collected data on the complete model of the OR and support analysis of the collected data via a proper set of data retrieval and visualization interfaces. Here, we introduced the OR-Use framework and demonstrated how the proposed architecture can address most of these requirements, as a usability support tool for the OR. Conducting more tests with different devices and providing a data mining interface to support the decision making process have to be the central aspects of future work.

References

1. Ardito, C., Costabile, F., De Marsico, M., Lanzilotti, R., Levialdi, S., Roselli, T., Rossano, V.: An approach to usability evaluation of e-learning applications. Univers. Access Inf. Soc. 4, 270–283 (2006)
2. AttrakDiff, http://www.attrakdiff.de/en/Home/
3. Au, F.T.W., Baker, S., Warren, I., Dobbie, G.: Automated usability testing framework. In: Ninth Australasian User Interface Conference, vol. 76, pp. 55–64. ACS, Wollongong (2008)
4. Bigdelou, A., Sterner, T., Wiesner, S., Wendler, T., Matthes, F., Navab, N.: OR Specific Domain Model for Usability Evaluations of Intra-operative Systems. In: Taylor, R.H., Yang, G.-Z. (eds.) IPCAI 2011. LNCS, vol. 6689, pp. 25–35. Springer, Heidelberg (2011)
5. Holm, R., Priglinger, M., Stauder, E., Volkert, J., Wagner, R.: Automatic data acquisition and visualization for usability evaluation of virtual reality systems. In: EUROGRAPHICS 2002. The Eurographics Association (2002)

6. Ivory, M.Y., Hearst, M.A.: The state of the art in automating usability evaluation of user interfaces. ACM Comput. Surv. 33, 470–516 (2001)
7. Liljegren, E.: Usability in a medical technology context assessment of methods for usability evaluation of medical equipment. Int. J. of Ind. Erg. 36(4), 345–352 (2006)
8. Morae, http://www.techsmith.com/morae.html
9. Neumuth, T., Durstewitz, N., Fischer, M., Strauss, G., Dietz, A., Meixensberger, J., Jannin, P., Cleary, K., Lemke, H.U., Burgert, O.: Structured recording of intraoperative surgical workflows. In: Society of Photo-Optical Instrumentation Engineers (SPIE) Conference Series, vol. 6145, pp. 54–65 (2006)
10. Nielsen, J.: Usability Engineering. Academic Press Inc., London (1993)
11. Strauss, G., Koulechov, K., Rttger, S., Bahner, J., Trantakis, C., Hofer, M., Korb, W., Burgert, O., Meixensberger, J., Manzey, D., Dietz, A., Lth, T.: Evaluation of a navigation system for ENT with surgical efficiency criteria. The Laryngoscope 116(4), 564–572 (2006)
12. Wachter, R.M.: The End of the Beginning: Patient Safety Five Years After 'To Err Is Human'. Health Affairs (2004)

Improving the Development of Surgical Skills with Virtual Fixtures in Simulation

Albert Hernansanz[1,2], Davide Zerbato[3], Lorenza Gasperotti[3],
Michele Scandola[3], Paolo Fiorini[3], and Alicia Casals[1,2]

[1] Institute for Bioengineering of Catalonia (IBEC)
[2] Technical University of Catalonia BarcelonaTech (UPC)
[3] Department of Computer Science, University of Verona

Abstract. This paper focuses on the use of virtual fixtures to improve the learning of basic skills for laparoscopic surgery. Five virtual fixtures are defined, integrated into a virtual surgical simulator and used to define an experimental setup based on a trajectory following task.

46 subjects among surgeons and residents underwent a training session based on the proposed setup. Their performance has been logged and used to identify the effect of virtual fixtures on the learning curve from the point of view of accuracy and completion time.

Virtual fixtures prove to be effective in improving the learning and affect differently accuracy and completion time. This suggests the possibility to tailor virtual fixtures on the specific task requirements.

1 Introduction

Surgeons training is mainly based on a Halstedian apprenticeship model [4] whereby residents learn by directly assisting an experienced surgeon during the intervention and slowly increase their hands-on experience over time. Considerable ethical, economic and legal problems affecting this approach led to the development of alternative tools to improve of laparoscopic and robotic surgical skills whose goal is to ensure surgeons proficiency before they start operating.

Basic abilities are prerequisites for the correct and safe performance of any surgical gesture and in particular for the execution of robotic surgery procedures. They allow the subject to cope with the perceptual abnormalities that characterize robotic surgery. Surgeons should undergo visuo-spatial and perceptual-motor abilities training to increase their proficiency in presence of indirect mapping between hands and robot and in absence of force feedback. A proper training of visuo-spatial skills allows the subject to redeem the lack of haptic information.

Virtual simulators demonstrated to effectively support the acquisition of the skills required by minimally invasive surgery outside the operating room in a safer, less stressing and cheapest way. Real time data recording constitutes a relevant advantage provided by those tools and makes their application in training and evaluation extremely valuable and effective.

The goal of this work is the assessment of assistive technologies in improving the development of basic skills in surgical training, following the Skill-Rule-Knowledge (SRK) taxonomy [7]. Five different assistance modalities have been

P. Abolmaesumi et al. (Eds.): IPCAI 2012, LNAI 7330, pp. 157–166, 2012.
© Springer-Verlag Berlin Heidelberg 2012

selected through the analysis of the state of the art and the observation of surgeons experience in the operating room and integrated into a surgical simulator. These assistive technologies have been parameterized by a single function to adapt their behavior to the task proposed in the experiment. A specific experimental design evaluated the improvement in the learning due to these aids.

Section 2 provides an overview of work related to the use assistive technologies in surgical tasks. Each individual aids extracted through the analysis of the state of the art is detailed in Section 3. Section 4 presents the integration of the virtual fixtures in the simulator and the experiment designed to identify assistance outcome. Experimental results are described and discussed in Section 5. Conclusions and future developments are proposed in Section 6.

2   Related Work

The design of different assistive technologies follows the SRK taxonomy proposed by Rasmussen in [7]. The theory distinguishes between skill- rule- and knowledge-based laparoscopic skills. Each behavioral level corresponds to a different degree of familiarity with the task to execute. By keeping into account this taxonomy it is possible to develop learning aids that are effective through the whole training process and to objectively evaluate them.

The skill based level (SBL) groups perceptual-motor and visuo-spatial skills. The skill-based behavior origins from sensory-motor informations, it is strongly automatized and temporally synchronic with the perception of environmental signals [10]. Number of errors and task completion time are the metrics most frequently considered in the evaluation of skill-based abilities. Previous work, based on the introduction of assistive aids in surgical training proves that the introduction of virtual fixtures (VF) in surgical training shorten the time required to develop SBL abilities [9]. These VF can be defined as a set of rules that modify the behavior of the telemanipulated devices in order to improve different aspects such as dexterity, accuracy or repeatability.

One of the most widely applied VF in surgical training is motion scaling (MS). The benefits of MS in robotic surgery is evaluated in [8], where different fixed scaling factors are applied to a tele-surgery system. The improvement in user performance is measured in terms of errors and completion time. The usefulness of virtual fixtures in user assistance is widely accepted and DaVinci surgical system integrates MS and allows the surgeon to set the scaling factor.

In [2] a study of the MS and tremor reduction benefits using the Zeus Surgical System is done. Subjects touch six different targets with an endoscopic tool with and without robotic assistance. When aid is enabled three different levels of motion scaling are used in addition to tremor filtering. Authors state that MS greatly improves accuracy whereas tremor filtering has limited effect.

In [5] pick-and-place tasks in micro-metric workspace are performed using three different modes: unassisted, hand held (with compliant robot) and autonomous. During the experiments fixed motion scaling is combined with a magnified vision on a Steady Hand robot and a LARS robot.

The integration of motion scaling and magnification is also studied in [1]. The paper states that MS reduces the errors when high magnification is used but, on the other hand, this increases the task completion time. Thus the authors suggest the need of trade off between motion scaling and magnification to optimize time and accuracy. Similarly, the work described in [6] deforms robot workspace to provide higher resolution on predefined region of interest: the scaling factor is a function of the distance between the Tool Center Point (TCP) and the target point. Authors also propose a vector-based approach, in which the scaling depends on the direction of motion.

During the initial phases of the training, the cognitive load experienced by the user may be considerably high as he/she has to acquire a relevant amount of information from the environment. By providing information through multiple sensorial modalities it is possible to reduce the cognitive load of the subject and thus ease the learning [11]. Assistive technologies have been applied in many different tasks and modalities, but at the best of author's knowledge, there is a lack in the comparison of virtual fixtures effects and in the evaluation of perceptual modalities for the improvement of the training in robotic surgery.

3   Virtual Fixtures

The analysis of the state of the art lead to the identification of five different assistance tools. Virtual fixtures differentiates for the modality used to convey information to the user and for the modification induced in the master/slave mapping. To isolate the effects of each fixture, all of them the have been defined and applied separately. A modulation function is introduced to control the behavior of the VFs, easing the comparison of the fixtures and allowing the complete control of all the VF through a reduced set of parameters whose effects are easy to understand and set up. All the VFs described in the following exploit the function to provide guidance to the user avoiding tight restriction on movements and leaving him/her the ultimate control over the TCP position.

The modulation function selected for all the fixtures is the five-parameter logistic function, f5PL [3] defined in (1), based on the basic sigmoid function

$$\text{f5PL}(x) = d + \frac{a - d}{(1 + (x/c)^b)^g} \tag{1}$$

where a and d are the expected value of f5PL at zero and at infinite respectively, b controls the slope of the curve between a and d, c is the mid-range concentration and g is the asymmetry factor.

Let $dist_{norm}$ indicates the distance between the target point and the device position normalized by the maximum allowed error. Three regions can be identified in the function domain. Close to the POI ($dist_{norm} \rightarrow 0$), the modulation has a constant value of a. This defines a region for dexterous work without disturbances due to VF. When the distance is near to its maximum ($dist_{norm} \rightarrow 1$) the modulation tends to b. The initial part of the task is performed in this region, where no changes on the modulation function are required. The two regions are

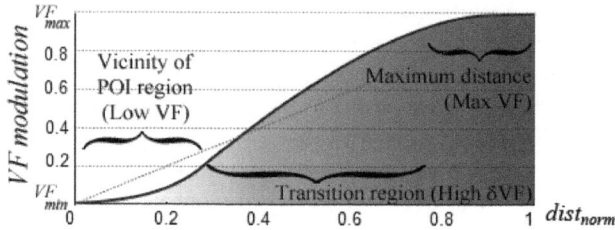

Fig. 1. f5PL modulation function applied to MS for point targeting task

linked by a transition zone that ensures smooth variations. In this zone the modulation varies quickly and the changes in VF's effects are easily noticed by the surgeon. Fig. 1 shows the modulation function and highlights the three regions.

Visual Guidance (VG) provides the surgeon with a guidance tool that acts through the visual sensory channel and originates a motor behavior. VG consists on a graphical representation of the minimum distance vector between the TCP and the goal point that provides surgeons with. information about the proximity of delicate regions and possible collisions while approaching the POI. Fig. (2) shows the VG used in trajectory following.

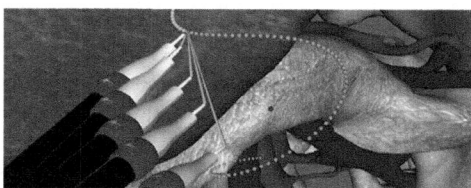

Fig. 2. Sequence of different tool positions and corresponding minimum distance vectors generated by the VG

Audio Guidance (AG) is the transposition of the VG to the auditive domain: errors are signaled to the user through sounds that may correct the motor behavior, helping the surgeon to keep the TCP close to the trajectory. Changes in the properties of the sound signal are controlled by the modulated distance between the tool and the goal point: when the error increases, the elapsed time between two consecutive sound signals decreases and the sample frequency increases. In presence of significative errors, the sound changes are easily perceived and provide a guidance effect.

Motion Scaling (MS) increases the accuracy of the surgeon by modifying the scaling factor between the master and the slave. In bilateral teleoperated systems, the motion of the slave depends on master device input, i.e. $X_S = f(X_M)$. Usually, f includes a fixed scale parameter, whereas MS provides a variable

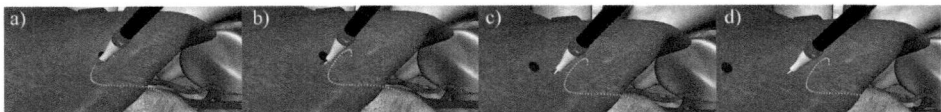

Fig. 3. Sequence of snapshots of the tool with the MS applied in trajectory following

vector-based scale parameter that is function of the error between the TCP and the POI. MS factor is computed and applied independently to each TCP component. Fig. 3 shows a set of snapshots of the application of the MS parameterized to follow a trajectory. The cone represents the position of the tool as if no motion scale was applied.

Magnification (Mag) provides the surgeon with an automated magnification and positioning of the endoscopic camera. This ensures that when the TCP is away from the target point the user has a wide view of the environment, whereas when the TCP is close to the target point a magnified view allows the user to perceive the fine details of the area of interest. Fig. 4 presents some screenshots of Mag: if the TCP is far from the POI, a general view of the scene is provided (Fig. 4.a). As the TCP gets closer to the POI the view is magnified (Fig. 4.b and Fig. 4.c) until the maximum magnification is applied (Fig. 4.d).

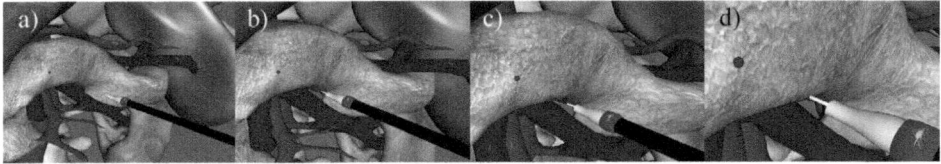

Fig. 4. Snapshots of the VA with the Mag enabled

Force Feedback (FF) guides the tool towards the POI with an attraction force. The direction of the applied force vector corresponds to the minimum distance vector from the TCP to the POI. The behavior of the attraction force follows the spring-damper model (2)

$$F = -Kd_{norm} - C\partial d_{norm}/\partial t. \tag{2}$$

The elastic and damping coefficients (K and C respectively) are the result of modulating two pre-defined coefficients, k and c, using d_{norm} as input parameter, $K = kf5PL(d_{norm})$ and $C = cf5PL(d_{norm})$. This modulation provides a non linearly-varying force that is negligible when the error is small and smoothly reaches the maximum when the error increases.

4   Experimental Design

To evaluate the effects of VFs in robotic surgery training they have been integrated into a virtual environment. The advantages of virtual over real environments are manifold: they allow the full control over the trials parameters and ensure repeatability and provide a portable and low cost setup.

The chosen virtual environment is based on the work described in [12] to which the reader is referred. It provides a reconstruction of abdominal anatomy in which the user can perform surgical tasks such as probing, grabbing, clamping or cutting. The whole simulation runs on a laptop equipped with a 17" monitor, user input and haptic rendering is handled by a Sensable PHANToM Omni. The experimental set up is depicted in Fig. 5.

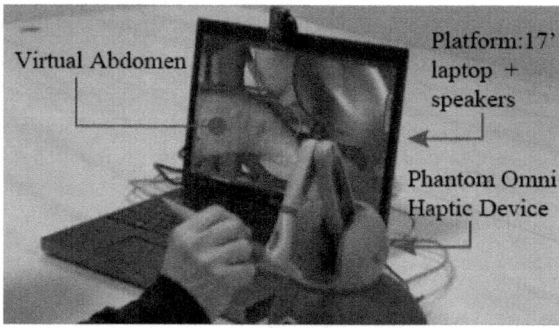

Fig. 5. The experimental setup

The integration of VFs into a virtual environment allows the development of the experiments required to analyze the effects of each VF individually. The designed task requires the user to follow different trajectories defined by 110 points by touching all the points in sequence with the TCP. The organs in the scene restrict tool movements, forcing the surgeon to avoid collisions and to deal with occlusions. The action of following a trajectory in a complex environment with regions to be avoided is a basic and recurrent gesture in many different procedures and it is not strictly related to a particular surgical field. Thus, the performance in trajectory following task can be a good measure of subjects manual dexterity. During the experiment the rendering of forces due to contacts with organs has been disabled to avoid interferences/overlap with VFs. This ensures the same base conditions for all the trials.

The evaluation of any fixture requires the assessment of subject's proficiency without VFs assistance. Thus the first part of the experiment identifies the subject base line performance with 3 VF-free trials. The second part proposes 5 blocks composed by 6 trials, all of them assisted by the same VF, followed by one VF free trial. During the five blocks, scheduled to cover all the considered VFs, the subject faces 6 different trajectories obtained by mirroring and rotating a single original path. This ensures that their difficulty is the same in terms of curvature and length and reduces any learning effect. The six trajectories are presented in a randomized order to avoid any facilitatory effect due to specific orientation sequence. On the contrary, all the VF-free trials are carried out on the same trajectory to exclude trajectory specific bias.

Before the experiment subjects are provided with a short introduction to the experiment goals, the virtual simulator capabilities and to VF. After the introduction, a questionnaire collects subject personal and experience data then the trials are proposed to the subject. Finally, a second questionnaire gets the subjective evaluation of each VF and possible suggestions.

Statistical analyses rely on the improvements in task accuracy and completion time due to virtual fixtures. The analyses isolate and verify the effects of each virtual fixture on the learning process and at identify the presence of significative differences between them. The learning curve is estimated by comparing only the set of VF-free trials, Repeated Measures Analysis of Variance (RM-ANOVA) and Tukey's Honestly Significant Difference (HSD) post-hoc test are applied on aggregated data.

5   Results

The experiment sample is composed by 46 subjects. 31 of them are surgeons and 15 residents with different background. Fig. 6 shows the composition of the sample by specialization (Fig. 6.a), experience in laparoscopy (Fig. 6.b) and experience with surgical simulators (Fig. 6.c) or in robotic surgery (Fig. 6.d).

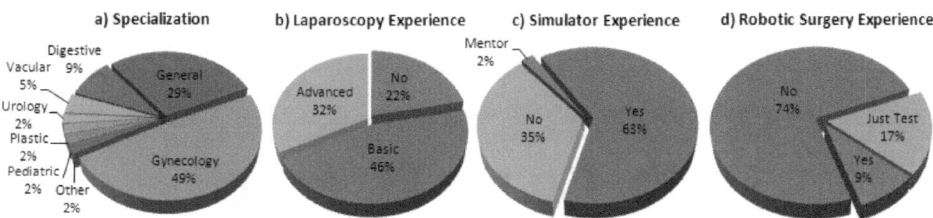

Fig. 6. Statistics of experiment population

At each temporal step k the system logs the position of the TCP $\mathbf{x}(k)$ and coordinates of the goal point $\mathbf{g}(k)$ on the trajectory, in addition, when the user passes through a trajectory point p the system stores the elapsed time since the beginning of the trial t_p. Since each trial has a different completion time and thus a different amount of sampled data, values logged during each trial have been aggregated to ensure the comparability of the results. For the i-th trajectory point of coordinates $\mathbf{p}_i$ the cumulative error e_i and the latency l_i are defined:

$$e_i = \sum_{j|\mathbf{p}_i=\mathbf{g}(j)} \|\mathbf{x}(j) - \mathbf{p}_i\|_1 \tag{3}$$

$$l_i = t_i - t_{1-i} \tag{4}$$

i.e. the total distance covered (measured with the Manhattan distance) and the time spent to move from the point to the next one.

The proposed experimental design includes two factors: virtual fixtures (6 levels, one for each VF plus the VF free scenario) and the trial number (8 levels: one for each VF free trial in the sequence). The analysis of the performance trend of the subjects evaluated during the whole experiment by the VF free trials and among each VF trials provides different results for the error measure and for the latency measure. The mean values of the cumulative error and the latency are shown in Fig. 7 and Fig. 8 respectively.

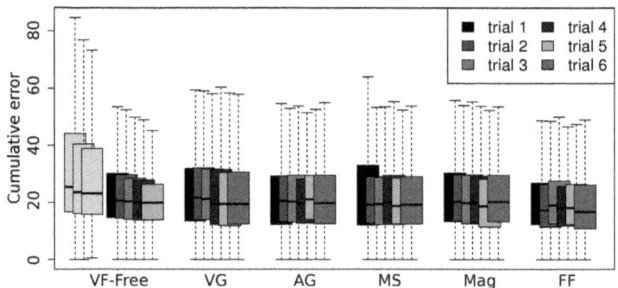

Fig. 7. Mean value and interquartile ranges (lower bound, first and third quartile, upper bound) for the cumulative error along trials

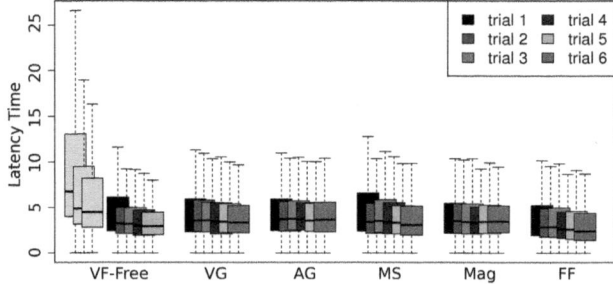

Fig. 8. Mean value and interquartile ranges (lower bound, first and third quartile, upper bound) for the latency along trials

The trend of the cumulative error for the VF free trials shows a considerable gap between the third and the fourth repetition. The gap between the trials then decreases significantly. The step in the cumulative error trend appears in correspondence with the first block of VF assisted trials after the three initial VF free repetitions. These results lead to the conclusion that the introduction of any virtual fixture strongly affects the user performance and that this effects continues even when the support of the VF is disabled. This analysis does not allow to identify the most effective VF, since their random presentation order drops the effect of VF factor. The trend of latency plots does not allow to assume any positive effect of VFs on the completion time. Together with the considerations provided for the cumulative error, this suggests that VFs are effective in increasing subject's accuracy but they do not increase the speed of user's motion.

RM-ANOVA applied to data collected during the VF assisted trials shows the statistical significance of the VF factor with a value of $F_{(5,98131)} = 35.030$, $p < 0.001$ for the cumulative error analysis and a value of $F_{(5,98131)} = 44.099$, $p < 0.001$ for the latency analysis. The effect of the trial factor is also significant for cumulative error $F_{(7,98131)} = 22.871$, $p < 0.001$ and latency $F_{(7,98131)} = 87.344$, $p < 0.001$. This proves that different VFs provide different effect on user performance. Tukey HSD test shows that FF is the most effective VF in reducing cumulative error but its effect is not significantly different from AG and MS. The same test on latency values shows that completion time is improved by Mag and that its effect is not significantly different from the one of AG.

6   Conclusions and Future Work

The work presented in this paper analyzes the effects of VFs on the learning of basic surgical skills in virtual training environments. Five different VFs have been integrated in a surgical simulator and proposed as training supports to surgeons and residents for a trajectory following task.

Data collected during the analysis highlight the positive influence of VFs on subjects' learning and allow the evaluation of the effectiveness of the proposed VFs in terms of cumulative error and latency reduction. The difference between the effects of VFs has been assessed by a RM-ANOVA. FF proves to be the most effective fixture in reducing the cumulative error, whereas Mag provides the strongest effect on the latency. Since in most surgical tasks accuracy has to be preferred over speed the outcome of this analysis suggests to focus training assistance on the FF and on the haptic channel on which FF relies. In addition, the positive effect of AG on both the evaluation parameters indicates that the audio channel can be effectively used to convey information to the user.

The proposed analysis will be extended to evaluate the performance of the subjects in presence of occlusions along the trajectory, thanks to the heterogeneous composition of the sample we will be able to evaluate the effect of subjects expertise on the performance. Moreover we will verify the effect of combining multiple VFs to increase the overall effect and evaluate the need for developing additional VFs to fit other tasks peculiarities.

Acknowledgments. This research was supported by SAFROS project (Patient safety in robotic surgery; http://www.safros.eu) which has received funding from the European Union Seventh Framework Programme (FP7/2007-2013) under grant agreement no 248960.

The authors wish to thank Ospedale Policlinico G.B. Rossi (Verona), Istituto Scientifico Universitario San Raffaele (Milano), Ospedale Policlinico Universitario di Padova, Consorci Sanitari de l'Anoia - Hospital d'Igualada, Hospital

Universitari Arnau de Vilanova (Lleida), Clinica de Ponent (Lleida), Hospital de la Santa Creu i Sant Pau (Barcelona), Hospital Universitari Vall d'Hebron (Barcelona) and Corporació Sanitària Parc Taulí (Sabadell) for the cooperation in data collection.

References

1. Cassilly, R., Diodato, M.D., Bottros, M., Damiano, R.J.: Optimizing motion scaling and magnification in robotic surgery. Surgery 136(2), 291–294 (2004)
2. Clayman, R.V.: Surgical robotics: impact of motion scaling on task performance. The Journal of Urology 174(3), 953 (2005)
3. Gottschalk, P.G., Dunn, J.R.: The five-parameter logistic: A characterization and comparison with the four-parameter logistic. Analytical Biochemistry 343(1), 54–65 (2005)
4. Halsted, W.: The training of the surgeon. Bullettin of the Johns Hopkins Hospital (1904)
5. Kumar, R., Goradia, T.M., Barnes, A.C., Jensen, P., Whitcomb, L.L., Stoianovici, D., Auer, L.M., Taylor, R.H.: Performance of Robotic Augmentation in Microsurgery-Scale Motions. In: Taylor, C., Colchester, A. (eds.) MICCAI 1999. LNCS, vol. 1679, pp. 1108–1115. Springer, Heidelberg (1999)
6. Munoz, L., Casals, A., Amat, J., Puig-Vidal, M., Samitier, J.: Improved afm scanning methodology with adaptation to the target shape. In: International Conference on Robotics and Automation, pp. 1529–1534 (April 2005)
7. Rasmussen, J.: Skills, rules, and knowledge; signals, signs, and symbols, and other distinctions in human performance models, pp. 291–300. IEEE Press, Piscataway (1987)
8. Salcudean, S.E., Ku, S., Bell, G.: Performance measurement in scaled teleoperation for microsurgery. In: Proceedings of the First Joint Conference on Computer Vision, Virtual Reality and Robotics in Medicine and Medial Robotics and Computer-Assisted Surgery, pp. 789–798. Springer, London (1997)
9. Wagner, C.R., Howe, R.D., Stylopoulos, N.: The role of force feedback in surgery: Analysis of blunt dissection. In: Proceedings of the 10th Symposium on Haptic Interfaces for Virtual Environment and Teleoperator Systems, HAPTICS 2002, p. 73. IEEE Computer Society, Washington, DC (2002)
10. Wentink, M., Stassen, L.P.S., Alwayn, I., Hosman, R.J.A.W., Stassen, H.G.: Rasmussen model of human behavior in laparoscopy training. Surgical Endoscopy 17, 1241–1246 (2003)
11. Wickens, C.: Processing resources and attention, p. 334. Taler & Francis, Ltd., Bristol (1991)
12. Zerbato, D., Baschirotto, D., Baschirotto, D., Botturi, D., Fiorini, P.: Gpu-based physical cut in interactive haptic simulations. International Journal of Computer Assisted Radiology and Surgery 6, 265–272 (2011)

Sparse Hidden Markov Models for Surgical Gesture Classification and Skill Evaluation

Lingling Tao[2], Ehsan Elhamifar[2],
Sanjeev Khudanpur[2], Gregory D. Hager[3], and René Vidal[1]

[1] BME
[2] CS
[3] ECE
Dept., Johns Hopkins University, Baltimore MD, 21218, USA

Abstract. We consider the problem of classifying surgical gestures and skill level in robotic surgical tasks. Prior work in this area models gestures as states of a hidden Markov model (HMM) whose observations are discrete, Gaussian or factor analyzed. While successful, these approaches are limited in expressive power due to the use of discrete or Gaussian observations. In this paper, we propose a new model called sparse HMMs whose observations are sparse linear combinations of elements from a dictionary of basic surgical motions. Given motion data from many surgeons with different skill levels, we propose an algorithm for learning a dictionary for each gesture together with an HMM grammar describing the transitions among different gestures. We then use these dictionaries and the grammar to represent and classify new motion data. Experiments on a database of surgical motions acquired with the da Vinci system show that our method performs on par with or better than state-of-the-art methods.This suggests that learning a grammar based on sparse motion dictionaries is important in gesture and skill classification.

Keywords: Surgical skill evaluation, surgical gesture classification, time series classification, sparse dictionary learning, hidden Markov models.

1 Introduction

Direct instruction by an expert is arguably the most effective means of learning the art of surgery. However, due to reductions in the amount of one-on-one teaching [1], an expert may not always be available to oversee and guide residents and fellows. Robotic surgery systems, such as the da Vinci robot, provide a well-instrumented, controlled laboratory for recording surgical performance. Such recordings can be used to model surgeon expertise and help understand how to reflect this expertise back upon students in the form of teaching and training.

Prior Work. One approach to modeling surgical expertise is to use global measurements of the task, such as the time to completion [2, 3], the speed and number of hand movements [2], the distance travelled [3], force and torque signatures [3–5], etc. These methods are generally easy to implement, but lack a detailed description of the surgical procedure. Another approach is to use statistical models to decompose a surgical task into a series of pre-defined surgical

P. Abolmaesumi et al. (Eds.): IPCAI 2012, LNAI 7330, pp. 167–177, 2012.

gestures or *surgemes* [6–11]. For example, in a suturing task, the surgemes can be 'insert a needle', 'grab a needle', 'position a needle', etc. Notice that these surgemes often appear in some pattern, e.g., one surgeme often follows another one, or several surgemes form a motif. This is analogous to what we see in natural language, where the grammar constrains the generation of words. In the case of surgery, however, we know neither the words nor the grammar. Thus, we need to develop algorithms for discovering the grammar and for classifying gestures and skill. Hidden Markov models (HMMs) provide an excellent framework for doing this. The simplest approach is to model each surgeme as the state of an HMM and to vector-quantize the observations from each surgeme into discrete symbols [6, 7]. Alternatively, one can model the observations from each surgeme using a Gaussian [8]. However, parameter learning may not be robust when the data is high-dimensional because of the large number of parameters to be estimated. To address this issue, [9] combines Gaussian HMMs (G-HMMs) with Linear Discriminant Analysis (LDA) [12], while [10] proposes several variations of HMMs, such as Factor Analyzed HMMs (FA-HMMs), and Switched Linear Dynamical Systems (SLDSs), which model the observations as being generated from a lower-dimensional latent space. However, the observation model is still Gaussian, which may not be rich enough to capture the variability of complex gestures. While one could use Gaussian mixture models (GMMs) [11] or mixtures of factor analyzers (MFAs) to describe more complex motions, this would again results in a large number of parameters to be estimated.

Paper Contributions. To achieve a richer observation model, without dramatically increasing the number of parameters to be estimated, in this paper we propose to use a sparse model as the HMM observation model. More specifically, we propose to model each observation as a sparse linear combination of elements from a dictionary of atomic surgical motions associated with a specific surgeme. Therefore, the observations from each surgeme live in a union of K-dimensional subspaces, one subspace per choice of K out of N atoms. While other models such as MFAs also represent the data with a union of subspaces, the number of parameters in our model is much smaller because we assume that the coefficients are sparse, and so only a few dictionary elements are used to represent a given observation. As a consequence, our observation model is more expressive than a Gaussian or a FA, but the number of parameters does not grow as rapidly as in the case of GMMs or MFAs. In principle, the parameters of the proposed sparse HMM can be learned using an expectation maximization algorithm. However, the expectation step cannot be computed in closed form. We thus propose an approximate parameter learning algorithm based on a sparse dictionary learning technique called KSVD [13]. We then show that surgeme classification can be done using the Viterbi algorithm [14], as in the case of G-HMMs. Experiments show that combining HMMs with sparse dictionary learning improves gesture and skill classification and achieves stable performance for various sparsity levels.

2   Sparse HMMs for Surgical Gesture and Skill Classification

Given a surgery trial $\{\boldsymbol{y}_t \in \mathbb{R}^D\}_{t=1}^T$, the goal of gesture classification is to assign a surgeme label $s_t \in \{1, \ldots, S\}$ to each frame, $\boldsymbol{y}_t$, while the goal of skill classification is to assign a skill level $z \in \{1, \ldots, L\}$ to the entire trial, $\{\boldsymbol{y}_t \in \mathbb{R}^D\}_{t=1}^T$. In this paper, we propose to model the trials using a sparse hidden Markov model (S-HMM). In this model, the surgeme label s_t is an unobserved hidden state, which is modeled as a Markov process characterized by the transition probability $q_{s's} = p(s_t = s | s_{t-1} = s')$. The observation at time t, $\boldsymbol{y}_t$, depends on the hidden state s_t via the emission probability density $p(\boldsymbol{y}_t | s_t)$.

In standard HMMs, which will be briefly reviewed in §2.1 and are illustrated in Fig. 1a, $p(\boldsymbol{y}_t | s_t)$ is assumed to be a Gaussian or a mixture of Gaussians. The parameters of this model can be learned using the Baum Welch algorithm [15], which is based on Expectation Maximization (EM). Given the model parameters, the hidden states can be inferred using the Viterbi algorithm.

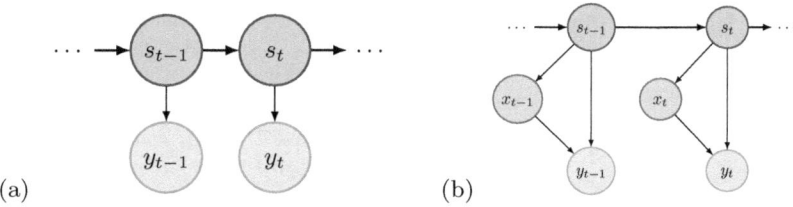

(a)   (b)

Fig. 1. Graphical models for standard HMMs (a) and HMMs with latent variables (b)

In the proposed S-HHMs, which will be discussed in §2.2 and are illustrated in Fig. 1b, the observation $\boldsymbol{y}_t$ is as a sparse linear combination of elements from a dictionary of motion words. Therefore, $\boldsymbol{y}_t$ also depends on another hidden variable, namely the sparse coefficients $\boldsymbol{x}_t$. In §2.3, we show that parameter learning for this model is more difficult than for G-HMMs, because the E-step cannot be computed in closed form. We thus propose an approximate learning approach based on sparse dictionary learning [13]. In §2.4, we show that surgeme classification can be done by combining a Viterbi-like algorithm with sparse coding [16, 17]. Finally, in §2.5 we show how to use S-HMMs for skill classification.

2.1   Prior Work on Gesture and Skill Classification Using HMMs

Much of the prior work on surgical gesture and skill classification uses HMMs [18, 6–11]. The main difference between different approaches is in how they model the emission probability density $p(\boldsymbol{y}_t | s_t)$. For example, [7] vector-quantizes the observations into discrete symbols, while [8] assumes a Gaussian distribution $p(\boldsymbol{y}_t | s_t = s) \equiv \mathcal{N}(\boldsymbol{u}_s, \boldsymbol{\Sigma}_s)$. These methods can leverage standard learning and inference algorithms. However, parameter learning is not robust with high-dimensional data due to the large number of parameters that need to be learned. Moreover, high-dimensional data often lie in low-dimensional subspaces, and this is not directly captured by a Gaussian distribution with an arbitrary covariance.

To address this problem, [9] uses a Gaussian model combined with LDA [12]. Alternatively, one can use Probabilistic PCA (PPCA) [19, 20] or Factor Analysis (FA) [21], as suggested in [10]. As illustrated in Fig. 1b, these models introduce a low-dimensional latent variable $x_t \in \mathbb{R}^d$, where $d \ll D$, and model the observations as $y_t = A_{s_t} x_t + u_{s_t} + e_t$, where $A_{s_t} \in \mathbb{R}^{D \times d}$, $u_{s_t} \in \mathbb{R}^D$, and x_t and e_t are independent Gaussians distributed as $\mathcal{N}(0, I)$ and $\mathcal{N}(0, \Sigma_{s_t})$, respectively. In PPCA, $\Sigma_{s_t} = \sigma_{s_t}^2 I$, while in FA, $\Sigma_{s_t} = \mathrm{diag}(\sigma_{1,s_t}^2, \ldots, \sigma_{D,s_t}^2)$. [10] proposes efficient learning and inference methods for this model and shows that using a low-dimensional model improves gesture classification results. This is possible, in part, because one can marginalize over the latent variables and obtain the emission probabilities in closed form as $p(y_t | s_t = s) \equiv \mathcal{N}(u_s, A_s A_s^T + \Sigma_s)$. Therefore, PPCA-HMMs and FA-HMMs are particular cases of G-HMMs.

In practice, modeling the data with a single subspace (as done by PPCA and FA) might not capture the distribution of the data for complex surgemes. To address this issue, one can use a mixture of low-dimensional subspaces, as proposed in [11]. This can be done by using MFAs, whose density can be written as:

$$p(y_t | s_t = s, x_t = x) \equiv \sum_{i=1}^{M} c_{si} \mathcal{N}(A_{si} x + u_{si}, \Sigma_{si}), \qquad (1)$$

where $c_{si} \in [0, 1]$ and $\sum_{i=1}^{M} c_{si} = 1$. In other words, c_{si} is the probability that y_t belongs to the i-th FA in the mixture. The drawbacks of using MFAs are that there are many parameters to be learned and that one needs to specify a priori the number of mixture components M and the dimension d of each FA.

2.2 Proposed Sparse Hidden Markov Model

In this section, we propose a new HMM that uses multiple subspaces to model the observations from each surgeme (thus being more general than single-subspace HMMs), but enforces sparsity constraints on the latent variables (thus rendering the parameter learning problem more robust). More specifically, we use recent advances in sparse dictionary learning and model the observation at time t as $y_t = D_{s_t} x_t + e_t$, where $D_{s_t} \in \mathbb{R}^{D \times N}$ is an over-complete dictionary ($D < N$), $x_t \in \mathbb{R}^N$ is a sparse latent variable, i.e., it has only a few nonzero entries, and e_t is independent Gaussian noise distributed as $\mathcal{N}(0, \sigma_{s_t}^2 I)$. As a result, the distribution of y_t given the latent variables is given by

$$p(y_t | s_t = s, x_t = x) \equiv \mathcal{N}(D_s x, \sigma_s^2 I). \qquad (2)$$

The key difference between our approach and MFAs in (1) is that, instead of fixing the number of mixture components M and their dimensions, we let the dictionary D_s be over-complete, but we choose a few columns of the dictionary using a sparse latent variable $\boldsymbol{x}_t$. This allows us to have an exponentially large number of subspaces to choose from and also to automatically pick the dimension of the low-dimensional subspace through the number of nonzero elements of $\boldsymbol{x}_t$.

To have a sparse latent variable, we use a Laplace prior on the distribution of $\boldsymbol{x}_t$ for each hidden state where

$$p(\boldsymbol{x}_t|s_t = s) \equiv \left(\frac{\lambda_s}{2}\right)^N \exp\left(-\lambda_s\|\boldsymbol{x}\|_1\right), \tag{3}$$

with a parameter $\lambda_s > 0$.

2.3   Parameter Learning in S-HMMs

Given N trials $\{\boldsymbol{y}_{1:T_j}^j\}_{j=1}^J$ from many surgeons with different skill levels and their surgeme labels $\{s_{1:T_j}^j\}_{j=1}^J$, our goal is to learn an S-HMM for these data. The parameters to be learned are the transition probabilities $Q = \{q_{s,s'}\}_{s,s'=1,\ldots,S}$ and the parameters for each surgeme model $\Theta_s = (\boldsymbol{D}_s, \sigma_s^2, \lambda_s)$, for $s = 1,\ldots,S$.

Since the surgeme labels are given, the transition probabilities can be directly computed from the frequency of surgeme transitions, and the remaining parameters can be learned separately from data corresponding to each surgeme s. Since $p(\boldsymbol{y}_t|s_t)$ depends on the hidden variable $\boldsymbol{x}_t$, we can use the EM algorithm to maximize the log-likelihood of the observations corresponding to surgeme s, $\mathcal{L}_{\Theta_s} = \sum_{j,t:s_t^j=s} \log p_{\Theta_s}(\boldsymbol{y}_t^j|s_t^j = s)$ w.r.t. the parameters Θ_s.

In the E-step we need to compute the expectation of the complete log-likelihood w.r.t. the posterior of $\boldsymbol{x}_t$, given the current parameters $\hat{\Theta}_s$, i.e.,

$$E_{\hat{\Theta}_s}(\mathcal{L}_{\Theta_s}) = \sum_{j,t:s_t^j=s} \int_{\boldsymbol{x}_t^j} \log p_{\Theta_s}(\boldsymbol{y}_t^j, \boldsymbol{x}_t^j|s_t^j = s) p_{\hat{\Theta}_s}(\boldsymbol{x}_t^j|\boldsymbol{y}_t^j, s_t^j = s) d\boldsymbol{x}_t^j. \tag{4}$$

However, this expression cannot be computed in closed form as in the case of G-HMMs. Following [22], we approximate the posterior as $p_{\hat{\Theta}_s}(\boldsymbol{x}_t^j|\boldsymbol{y}_t^j, s_t^j = s) = \delta(\hat{\boldsymbol{x}}_t^j)$, where $\hat{\boldsymbol{x}}_t^j = \arg\max_{\boldsymbol{x}} p_{\hat{\Theta}_s}(\boldsymbol{x}|\boldsymbol{y}_t^j, s_t^j = s) = \arg\max_{\boldsymbol{x}} p_{\hat{\Theta}_s}(\boldsymbol{y}_t^j|\boldsymbol{x}, s_t^j = s) p_{\hat{\Theta}_s}(\boldsymbol{x}|s_t^j = s)$. Therefore, the E-step reduces to the following ℓ_1-minimization problem

$$\hat{\boldsymbol{x}}_t^j = \arg\min_{\boldsymbol{x}} \hat{\lambda}_s\|\boldsymbol{x}\|_1 + \frac{1}{2\hat{\sigma}_s^2}\|\boldsymbol{y}_t^j - \hat{\boldsymbol{D}}_s\boldsymbol{x}\|^2, \tag{5}$$

which can be solved using a sparse coding algorithm such as Basis Pursuit [16]. With this approximation, we obtain the following approximate expectation

$$E_{\hat{\Theta}_s}(\mathcal{L}_{\Theta_s}) \approx \sum_{j,t:s_t^j=s} \log\left(p_{\Theta_s}(\boldsymbol{y}_t^j, \hat{\boldsymbol{x}}_t^j|s_t^j = s)\right) = \sum_{j,t:s_t^j=s} \log\left(p_{\Theta_s}(\boldsymbol{y}_t^j|\hat{\boldsymbol{x}}_t^j, s_t^j = s) p_{\Theta_s}(\hat{\boldsymbol{x}}_t^j|s_t^j = s)\right)$$

$$= \sum_{j,t:s_t^j=s} -\lambda_s\|\hat{\boldsymbol{x}}_t^j\|_1 - \frac{1}{2\sigma_s^2}\|\boldsymbol{y}_t^j - \boldsymbol{D}_s\hat{\boldsymbol{x}}_t^j\|_2^2 + N\log(\frac{\lambda_s}{2}) - \frac{D}{2}\log(2\pi\sigma_s^2). \tag{6}$$

In the M-step we need to maximize the above quantity w.r.t. Θ_s, which gives:

$$\hat{\boldsymbol{D}}_s = \sum_{j,t:s_t^j=s} \boldsymbol{y}_t^j\hat{\boldsymbol{x}}_t^{jT}\left(\sum_{j,t:s_t^j=s} \hat{\boldsymbol{x}}_t^j\hat{\boldsymbol{x}}_t^{jT}\right)^{-1}, \hat{\lambda}_s = \frac{\sum_{j,t:s_t^j=s} N}{\sum_{j,t:s_t^j=s} \|\hat{\boldsymbol{x}}_t^j\|_1}, \hat{\sigma}_s^2 = \frac{\sum_{j,t:s_t^j=s} \|\boldsymbol{y}_t^j - \hat{\boldsymbol{D}}_s\hat{\boldsymbol{x}}_t^j\|_2^2}{\sum_{j,t:s_t^j=s} D}. \tag{7}$$

Interestingly, the above approximate EM algorithm involves an E-step where the MAP estimate of x_t^j is calculated given $\hat{D}_s$ and an M-step where the dictionary D_s is updated based on $\hat{x}_t^j$. This is analogous to the method of optimal directions (MOD) in sparse dictionary learning, which alternates between finding the sparse coefficients and updating the dictionary [23]. This opens the door to using faster and more accurate sparse dictionary learning methods that update x_t^j and D_s jointly. One such algorithm is KSVD [13], which uses the ℓ_0-semi-norm instead of the ℓ_1-norm in the cost function. Since λ_s and σ_s^2 are not involved in KSVD, one can compute them afterwards by cross validation. We call this approximate learning method KSVD-HMM, and this is our method of choice.

2.4   Surgeme Classification Using S-HMMs

Given a trial $\{y_t\}_{t=1}^T$ and the S-HMM parameters $q_{s,s'}$ and Θ_s, $s, s' = 1, \ldots, S$, our goal is to infer the sequence of surgeme labels $\{s_t\}_{t=1}^T$. In standard HMMs this can be done by the Viterbi algorithm [14], where one maximizes the joint probability of the hidden states and the observations

$$(\hat{s}_{1:T}) = \operatorname{argmax} p(s_{1:T}|y_{1:T}) = \operatorname{argmax} p(s_{1:T}, y_{1:T}). \tag{8}$$

However, unlike the Gaussian, PPCA and FA models discussed in §2.1, the marginal probability $p(y_t|s_t)$ cannot be computed in closed form because x_t has a Laplace distribution. Nonetheless, in this section we show that the inference problem can still be solved using a dynamic programming approach. More specifically, we can write the following recursion

$$
\begin{aligned}
\alpha_t(s, x) &\triangleq \max_{s_{1:t-1}, x_{1:t-1}} p(s_{1:t-1}, x_{1:t-1}, s_t = s, x_t = x, y_{1:t}) \\
&= \max_{s', x'} \{ \max_{s_{1:t-2}, x_{1:t-2}} p(s_{1:t-2}, x_{1:t-2}, s_{t-1} = s', x_{t-1} = x', s_t = s, x_t = x, y_{1:t}) \} \\
&= \max_{s', x'} \{ \max_{s_{1:t-2}, x_{1:t-2}} p(y_t|x_t = x, s_t = s) \cdot p(x_t = x|s_t = s) \cdot q_{s', s} \\
&\qquad\qquad \cdot p(s_{1:t-2}, x_{1:t-2}, s_{t-1} = s', x_{t-1} = x', y_{1:t-1}) \} \\
&= p(y_t|x_t = x, s_t = s) \cdot p(x_t = x|s_t = s) \cdot \max_{s', x'} \{ q_{s', s} \cdot \alpha_{t-1}(s', x') \}. \tag{9}
\end{aligned}
$$

From the last equality, one can see that the value of x_t only affects the first two probabilities and has no influence on the last term. Now, since the number of states S is finite, for each s we can find the $\hat{x}_s$ that maximizes $p(y_t|x, s)p(x|s)$. That is, $\hat{x}_s = \operatorname{argmin}_x \lambda_s \|x\|_1 + \frac{1}{2\sigma_s^2} \|y_t - D_s x\|^2$, which can be found using Basis Pursuit [16] or Orthogonal Matching Pursuit (OMP) [17]. Since the learning algorithm uses KSVD, which in turn uses OMP, we also use OMP here.

2.5   Skill Classification Using S-HMMs

For skill classification, we model the data from different skill levels with different S-HMMs and classify a new trial by finding the model that gives the highest log-likelihood. More specifically, for each expertise level, we learn an S-HMM using

KSVD-HMM, the approximate learning algorithm described in §2.3. This gives us three models, $\mathcal{M}_e$, $\mathcal{M}_i$ and $\mathcal{M}_n$ corresponding to expert, intermediate and novice. Given a test trial $\{\boldsymbol{y}_t \in \mathbb{R}^D\}_{t=1}^T$, the skill level z is given by:

$$\hat{z} = \arg\max_{z \in \{e,i,n\}} p(\boldsymbol{y}_{1:T}, \boldsymbol{x}_{1:T}, s_{1:T} | \mathcal{M}_z). \qquad (10)$$

3   Experiments

Dataset Description. To evaluate the proposed KSVD-HMM approach for surgeme classification and to compare it with other state-of-the-art methods, we use the California dataset described in [7, 24, 25]. The dataset is acquired with the da Vinci surgical robot, which provides both kinematic data and high-resolution video data. For the experiments below, we use the kinematic data which consists of 78 variables describing the motion (velocity, rotation angle, position, etc.) of the master and slave robots. The dataset consists of 39, 26 and 36 trials, respectively, from three different tasks: suturing, needle passing and knot tying. Each task is performed by 8 surgeons of three expertise levels: expert, intermediate and novice. Typically each surgeon has around of $3 - 5$ trials for each task.

According to the definition of surgemes in [24], as listed in Fig. 2a, each of the trials is manually segmented into a sequence of surgemes, and the surgeme labels provide us the ground truth for surgeme classification. Each time series data consists, in general, of 11 different surgemes, as shown in Fig. 2b.

Experiment Setup. We create two different test setups. Setup 1 is the *leave-one-supertrial-out* setup, where we leave one trial from each one of the users out for testing, and use the remaining trials for training. Setup 2 is the *leave-one-user-out* setup, where we leave all the trials from one user out for testing and use the remaining trials for training.

0. Idle motion
1. Reach for needle
2. Position needle
3. Insert needle / push needle through tissue
4. Move to middle with needle (left hand)
5. Move to middle with needle (right hand)
6. Pull suture with left hand
7. Pull suture with right hand
8. Orienting needle with two hands
9. Right hand assisting left while pulling suture
10. Loosen more suture
11. End of trial

(a)

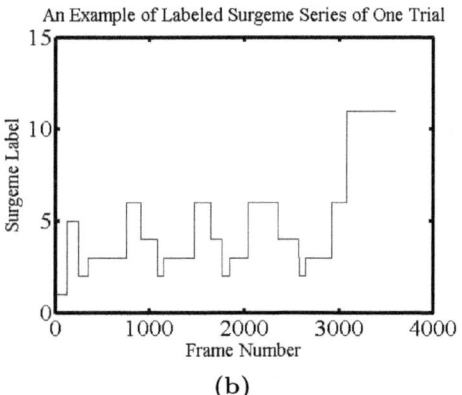

(b)

Fig. 2. List of surgemes (a) and sample surgeme time series (b)

Table 1. Best surgeme classification percentages obtained by different methods

		MFA-HMM	KSVD-HMM	FA-HMM(1)	SLDS(1)	FA-HMM(3)	HLDA-HMM	SLDS(3)
SU	Setup 1	76.4	**81.1**	70.2	74.8	78.2	74.1	80.8
	Setup 2	59.8	**67.8**	N/A	N/A	57.2	N/A	67.1
NP	Setup 1	74.2	76.1	64.3	72.3	71.0	65.0	**77.6**
	Setup 2	46.6	59.3	N/A	N/A	42.7	N/A	**60.0**
KT	Setup 1	76.5	82.6	77.1	78.5	**82.8**	79.9	82.0
	Setup 2	65.1	65.7	N/A	N/A	**67.0**	N/A	66.0

Surgeme Classification. We evaluate the surgeme classification performance of KSVD-HMM and compare it to that of MFA-HMM on three datasets. For KSVD-HMM we vary the sparsity level K and for MFA-HMM we vary the number of subspaces M and the dimensions d. The parameters σ and λ in KSVD-HMM are obtained by cross validation. The best results for each method using each of the two setups are shown in Table 1. We also compare our results to those in [10] for FA-HMM, HLDA-HMM, and SLDS.

Notice that in [10], each surgeme can be represented by 1 state HMM, or by a left-to-right HMM with 3 states. The first case is analogous to our model of one state per surgeme. The second case corresponds to a more sophisticated method in which surgemes are further decomposed into smaller components. The numbers 1 and 3 in parentheses after FA-HMM and SLDS indicate the number of HMM states used by [10] to represent each surgeme. We can see from Table 1 that, for suturing and setup 2 of knot tying task, KSVD-HMM outperforms even a more sophisticated 3-state HMM model, or 3-state SLDS model where both latent variables at time t depend on the latent variables at time $t-1$. For the other tasks, KSVD-HMM performs slightly worse than the 3-state SLDS, but is still better than any 1-state HMM model based on Gaussian models or SLDS. Overall, the proposed KSVD-HMM method performs on par with or better than state-of-the-art techniques.

Notice also that the performance of all methods decreases from setup 1 to setup 2. This is because in setup 2 all the trials from the same surgeon are excluded, which makes the classification problem more challenging because we only use the trials of the other surgeons.

Fig. 3 shows the effect of changing the parameters of each dictionary learning algorithm on the classification performance. From the plots in Fig. 3 we can see that the classification rates of MFA-HMM for different values of $M = 1, 5, 10, 15, 20$ and $d = 5, 10$ are in general lower than those of KSVD-HMM. Also note that for KSVD-HMM, the classification rates do not change much as we change the sparsity level $K = 3, 5, 7, 9, 11, 13, 15$. Thus, KSVD-HMM is less dependent on model selection than MFA-HMM, which makes it more favorable for classification using dictionary learning algorithms.

Skill Classification. We now evaluate the skill classification performance of KSVD-HMM and compare it to that of MFA-HMM. Table 2 shows the best classification results achieved by KSVD-HMM and MFA-HMM. For setup 1, where we have different data from the same user in both training and testing, KSVD-HMM performs clearly better than MFA-HMM. Notice also that for setup 2,

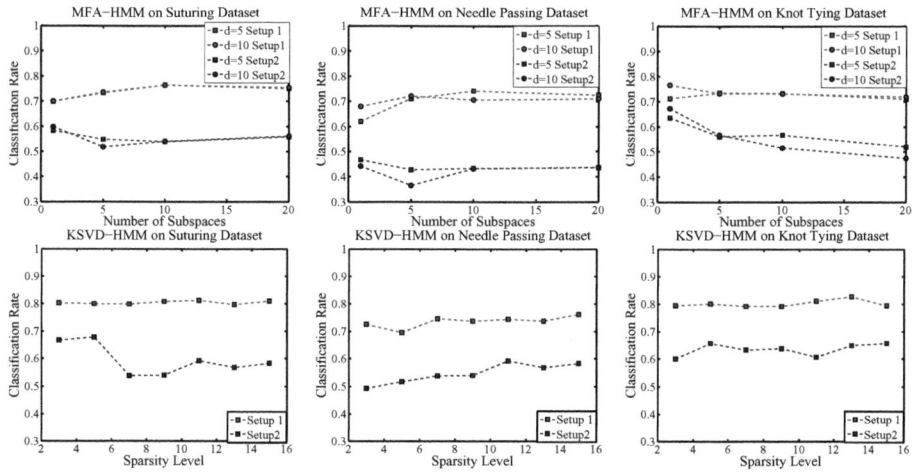

Fig. 3. Top: Surgeme classification rates of MFA-HMM as a function of the number of subspaces M and the subspace dimension d. Bottom: Surgeme classification results of KSVD-HMM as a function of the sparsity level K. Both methods are evaluated on three surgery tasks: suturing, needle passing and knot tying.

Table 2. Best skill classification percentages obtained by MFA-HMM and KSVD-HMM

	Suturing		Needle Passing		Knot Tying	
Setup	MFA-HMM	KSVD-HMM	MFA-HMM	KSVD-HMM	MFA-HMM	KSVD-HMM
Setup 1	92.3	97.4	76.9	96.2	86.1	94.4
Setup 2	38.5	59.0	46.2	26.9	44.4	58.3

where we exclude the trials of the same surgeon, we obtain much lower classification rates than for setup 1. In addition to the fact that we have excluded the trials of the same surgeon, another reason for this drop is the relatively small number of overall training data in the dataset, which does not allow us to capture well a specific skill level. For example, in the suturing data, we only have two experts, two intermediates and four novices. We are currently collecting larger datasets to be able to better evaluate the sensitivity of different methods.

4 Conclusion

We have proposed a new model called sparse HMMs for the classification of gestures and skill in surgical tasks. In this model, the observations are expressed as linear combinations of elements from a dictionary with sparse coefficients. The experiments show that the proposed methods achieve stable performance for various sparsity levels and perform on par with or better than the state of the art. Future work involves evaluation of the proposed methods on larger datasets.

Acknowledgment. This project was supported by grants NSF 0931805 and NSF 0941362. The authors thank Carol Reiley for providing the annotated dataset, and Balakrishnan Varadarajan for numerous discussions on the subject.

References

1. Barden, C., Specht, M., McCarter, M., Daly, J., Fahey, T.: Effects of limited work hours on surgical training. Obstetrical & Gynecological Survey 58(4), 244–245 (2003)
2. Datta, V., Mackay, S., Mandalia, M., Darzi, A.: The use of electromagnetic motion tracking analysis to objectively measure open surgical skill in laboratory-based model. Journal of the American College of Surgery 193, 479–485 (2001)
3. Judkins, T., Oleynikov, D., Stergiou, N.: Objective evaluation of expert and novice performance during robotic surgical training tasks. Surgical Endoscopy 1(4) (2008)
4. Richards, C., Rosen, J., Hannaford, B., Pellegrini, C., Sinanan, M.: Skills evaluation in minimally invasive surgery using force/torque signatures. Surgical Endoscopy 14, 791–798 (2000)
5. Yamauchi, Y., Yamashita, J., Morikawa, O., Hashimoto, R., Mochimaru, M., Fukui, Y., Uno, H., Yokoyama, K.: Surgical Skill Evaluation by Force Data for Endoscopic Sinus Surgery Training System. In: Dohi, T., Kikinis, R. (eds.) MICCAI 2002. LNCS, vol. 2488, pp. 44–51. Springer, Heidelberg (2002)
6. Rosen, J., Hannaford, B., Richards, C., Sinanan, M.: Markov modeling of minimally invasive surgery based on tool/tissue interaction and force/torque signatures for evaluating surgical skills. IEEE Trans. Biomedical Eng. 48(5), 579–591 (2001)
7. Reiley, C.E., Hager, G.D.: Task versus Subtask Surgical Skill Evaluation of Robotic Minimally Invasive Surgery. In: Yang, G.-Z., Hawkes, D., Rueckert, D., Noble, A., Taylor, C. (eds.) MICCAI 2009, Part I. LNCS, vol. 5761, pp. 435–442. Springer, Heidelberg (2009)
8. Rosen, J., Solazzo, M., Hannaford, B., Sinanan, M.: Task decomposition of laparoscopic surgery for objective evaluation of surgical residents' learning curve using hidden Markov model. Computer Aided Surgery 7(1), 49–61 (2002)
9. Varadarajan, B., Reiley, C., Lin, H., Khudanpur, S., Hager, G.: Data-Derived Models for Segmentation with Application to Surgical Assessment and Training. In: Yang, G.-Z., Hawkes, D., Rueckert, D., Noble, A., Taylor, C. (eds.) MICCAI 2009, Part I. LNCS, vol. 5761, pp. 426–434. Springer, Heidelberg (2009)
10. Varadarajan, B.: Learning and Inference Algorithms for Dynamical System Models of Dextrous Motion. PhD thesis, Johns Hopkins University (2011)
11. Leong, J.J.H., Nicolaou, M., Atallah, L., Mylonas, G.P., Darzi, A.W., Yang, G.-Z.: HMM Assessment of Quality of Movement Trajectory in Laparoscopic Surgery. In: Larsen, R., Nielsen, M., Sporring, J. (eds.) MICCAI 2006. LNCS, vol. 4190, pp. 752–759. Springer, Heidelberg (2006)
12. Lin, H.C., Shafran, I., Murphy, T.E., Okamura, A.M., Yuh, D.D., Hager, G.D.: Automatic Detection and Segmentation of Robot-Assisted Surgical Motions. In: Duncan, J.S., Gerig, G. (eds.) MICCAI 2005. LNCS, vol. 3749, pp. 802–810. Springer, Heidelberg (2005)
13. Aharon, M., Elad, M., Bruckstein, A.M.: K-SVD: An algorithm for designing overcomplete dictionaries for sparse representation. IEEE Trans. on Signal Processing 54(11), 4311–4322 (2006)
14. Forney Jr., G.D.: The Viterbi algorithm. Proceedings of the IEEE 61(3) (1973)
15. Baum, L.E., Petrie, T., Soules, G., Weiss, N.: A maximization technique occurring in the statistical analysis of probabilistic functions of Markov chains. Ann. Math. Statist. 41(1), 164–171 (1970)
16. Chen, S.S., Donoho, D.L., Saunders, M.A.: Atomic decomposition by basis pursuit. SIAM J. Sci. Comput. 20, 33–61 (1998)

17. Tropp, J.A., Gilbert, A.C.: Signal recovery from random measurements via orthogonal matching pursuit. IEEE Trans. on Information Theory 53(12), 4655–4666 (2007)
18. Dosis, A., Bello, F., Gillies, D., Undre, S., Aggarwal, R., Darzi, A.: Laparoscopic task recognition using hidden markov models. Studies in Health Technology and Informatics 111, 115–122 (2005)
19. Tipping, M., Bishop, C.: Probabilistic principal component analysis. Journal of the Royal Statistical Society 61(3), 611–622 (1999)
20. Tipping, M., Bishop, C.: Mixtures of probabilistic principal component analyzers. Neural Computation 11(2), 443–482 (1999)
21. McLachlan, G.J., Peel, D., R.W.B.: Modelling high-dimensional data by mixture of factor analyzers. Computational Statistics and Data Analysis 41, 379–388 (2003)
22. Olshausen, B.A., Field, B.J.: Sparse coding with an overcomplete basis set: a strategy employed by V1? Vision Research (1997)
23. Engan, K., Aase, S.O., Husoy, J.H.: Method of optimal directions for frame design. In: IEEE International Conference on Acoustics, Speech, and Signal Processing (1999)
24. Reiley, C.E., Lin, H.C., Varadarajan, B., Vagolgyi, B., Khudanpur, S., Yuh, D.D., Hager, G.D.: Automatic recognition of surgical motions using statistical modeling for capturing variability. In: Medicine Meets Virtual Reality, pp. 396–401 (2008)
25. Lin, H.: Structure in Surgical Motion. PhD thesis. Johns Hopkins University (2010)

Author Index